YOU MAY DIE EARLIER
WITHOUT KNOWING THIS

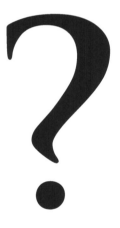

YOU MAY DIE EARLIER WITHOUT KNOWING THIS

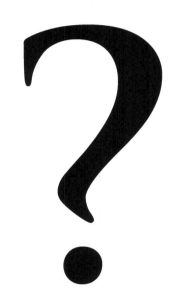

CHAN HUR

authorHOUSE®

AuthorHouse™
1663 Liberty Drive
Bloomington, IN 47403
www.authorhouse.com
Phone: 1-800-839-8640

Published by AuthorHouse   05/31/2013

ISBN: 978-1-4817-5498-9 (sc)
ISBN: 978-1-4817-5497-2 (e)

Library of Congress Control Number: 2013909422

CONTENTS

Introduction

I want to receive the Nobel Prize.

Half of the population would take on cancer by the year 2050. Even it is possible to prevent cancer, most don't know the fact and truth of the cancer. As we don't know where the cancers come from, we don't know how to prevent cancer. We are on stage just touching the surface, not on the core.

I really would like to receive the Nobel Prize. The reason is simple. If general public are aware of this information on this book and practice, cancer can be prevented easily. Even though I pass this information to my every patient in my clinic, how many can I let know this information? However if I receive Novel Prize, so many will get right information and be able to practice to prevent cancer. If everyone practice this information, the occurrence rate of cancer will be down substantially and the money that would be saved unimaginable. Of course many will not suffer with physical and emotional pain from cancer.

Hypertension and diabetes are no exception. More than half who are older than 60 years old suffer with hypertension. More than 25% suffer with diabetes over 60 years. The current medical system is concentrated on relieving only symptoms, not on the original cause. What a wasteful method! I believe there is much better way to get out of this trap at less cost.

I want a world where the common sense would be believed.

Yin Yang = superstitions?

Before I become an acupuncturist, I understood yin and yang are words representing the superstition. I also have considered this way in the name of science.

The general public does not know the meaning of yin and yang. They think yin and yang as a superstition. It may be a tool for the fortune teller and considered as a basic view for horoscope. Schools don't teach that yin-yang and the five elements are the moving force of universe for the daily life. Most don't know the meaning of even the calendar week.

As western medicine has been developed in the West, everything must be interpreted by science. The lack of statistics is considered unscientific even though it is a common sense. There is no exception on medicines, either.

Most blood tests are not able to detect many symptoms until blood vessels are clogged up to 70%. The accuracy is only 30%. The question is whether we can treat all 30%. Moreover it is not. We have to understand the frustration of many patients who begin to feel with modern medical treatments. Let us assume we may be able to treat two thirds of 30% and one thirds is not treatable. The conclusion is we don't know 80%. We just ignore this common sense.

What do we study to learn the human body at school? We have learned chromosomes which are XX for woman and XY for man in the study of biology. Even though we learn intellectually, the reality is that most general public doesn't need this information in the real world.

The thinking and meditation in most academic fields have been developed in the East. For example, the amount of blood during periods is determined to the supply of nutrients for the fetus. As soon as the umbilical cord is cut, the nutrient for the baby is changed into milk. This means less menstrual amount will lead less nutrients for the fetus and less milk for the baby. When I advise female this information, most answer that they don't know the importance of menstrual amount.

We also learn the importance of endorphin. Some claim its effectiveness is better than any pain medicine, so we have to laugh all the time. Here is my question. What about insulin, estrogen, progesterone and testosterone? Don't we need those? As we emphasize one small fact, the modern medicines are bruised, but most don't realize this fact.

Feeling pain or discomfort, even though all tests are negative

Many patients go to doctors as they feel their body is not normal. After the basic blood tests as well as various X-ray and MRI etc., many receive everything is normal. I am definitely sick, but tests show normal. How can we explain? It is called malingered sometimes. This makes us crazy. Someone may remember that when they see doctors, doctors told patients have neurogenic function issue 30-40 years ago. When my mother or other elders went the hospital, they heard the symptom was due to abnormal neurogenic function.

This abnormal neurogenic function has been changed into hypertensive stress since 20 years ago. A lot of people who read this would agree on me. Many patients are diagnosed by an autoimmune disease these days. All explanations mean current tests can't detect the real issues, in another words doctors don't know the reason either.

One nurse's story

A young nurse came with her mother. As she is a registered nurse and has a health insurance, she has done all kinds of tests known to her. All tests' results were negative. She complained her waist is always heavy and painful. So I answered the test result was wrong. But she told me as she is a nurse and capable to interpret, she reviewed all tests and confirmed negative. I told her again in this case even if you are not really sick, you feel sick to get an attention from someone or are lying you are sick. She became speechless and said she came here as she is really sick As far as I am concerned, the test results are wrong. She asked me again what went wrong about all knowledge she has learned for 4 years. So I answered her. All examination methods are created by man-made, not by almighty Creator. Why do you believe 100% for man-made? She agreed a little by that. So I explained as follows.

It is true that test methods have developed so greatly. Cancer had been checked by X-ray which is an only tool in the past. If the size was more than 30mm, medical people judged it as a cancer. If the size is less than 30mm, it was difficult to judge. Due to the great development we can judge easily if the size more than 5mm. However we still can't find if the size is less than 5mm. Can we find 1mm or 0.1mm? Of course we can't. She now nods and agrees what I explained. She asked a question that if I get a treatment by your way, this pain can be treated. I can't guarantee that, but I have never failed that kind of pain treatment. She decided to get my acupuncture treatment. After 30 minutes of treatment, I asked her to get up and move the waist. She moved the waist couple of times and reported the pain is gone. Her mother asked her "Are you sure the pain is gone?" She answered "this is amazing and marvelous". Her mother also delighted and laughed.

THE PAIN WE FEEL

According to western medicine there is almost no hindrance for blood to pass through until 70% of the blood vessels are clogged. This means we can say when we have already felt the pain, the state is already 70% clogged. Another fact is test results may not be shown until 50-70% clogging.

Kidney glomeruli filter waste products and send to the urinary bladder. When we can't urinate for one week, we may not live. However until 70% of glomerular are clogged, there is almost no interfere for urinations. This doesn't mean kidney has no problems on vessels or glomeruli

As I do not know how to inspect vessels or glomeruli, I don't know how accurate the number of 50-70% is. However I don't believe the inspection methods are 100% exact.

Even though this is a reality, the majority of patients believe doctors unconditionally.

What about the liver? The liver is called as a silent organ. This is well known to the public, too. Some say even 80% of failure of liver doesn't feel any awareness.

50% OF YIN DEPLETION ON FORTIES

Eastern medicine encyclopedia(東醫寶鑑) is very valuable book to acupuncturists. This book claims when human beings reach 50 years old, 50% of yin is consumed. If the life span is 100years, 50years are just the half. This means the capability of health remains the half. Although there is no way to prove scientifically, this really convinces us by common sense. When the time passes by we are getting old, it is just like using the machine for a long time means machine's life tearing down.

The start of the disease begins with the liver. The first one of four seasons comes from the spring and the next is summer, fall and winter. The same theory is birth, growth, harvest and storage or hiding. The lifespan also comes puberty, adulthood, middle age and the old age. In this context the liver is related with the spring, so we can say the beginning of the disease starts from the liver. However we don't feel the pain until the liver is damaged by 70-80%.

ORIENTAL HERB AND LIVER

Many people worry liver may fail out due to taking herb. There was a report that an acupuncturist in U.S.A. was sued a few years ago as the liver of a patient went bad suddenly from fine function after taking the herb by a few medical doctors of the patient. This report didn't mention the age or symptom of the patient at all. This report had been a big hit to other oriental clinic even though they are not related with that patient.

Western medicine calls all medicines are the poison. This is the concept of western medicine. However oriental medicine refrain the use of the word—ALL As I mention in this book even cigarettes are good in some cases. Based on this, rather getting worse with oriental herbal medicine it may improve liver function. In reality I treat hepatitis C successfully and even cirrhosis 4th stage with oriental herbal medicine. The formula used on was Tonify the Liver Decoction meaning this formula that tonifies the liver. Hepatitis C was treated by removing the liver heat rather caused by viral hepatitis. Virus may not like the coldness in my opinion.

CONCLUSION

It depends on how we think. We should discard bias western diagnose is 100% right and oriental herbal medication damage the liver. When there is no specific diagnostic result, there may be an answer somewhere. Heaven helps those who help themselves. When you seek you may find the answer. Please give up the idea that all diagnostic results are right. How do human beings know and understand everything by 100%?

CAUSES OF DISEASES

Old sage said there are only 3 causes of diseases. The first is the external, the second is the internal and the third is something that doesn't belong to the external and the internal. When you think about this seriously, this is well described just like hitting the bull's eye.

1. EXTERNAL CAUSE

This is due to seasons. These are wind, hot, dampness, dryness, and cold. When these are related with seasons, these are spring, summer, late summer, fall and winter. Simply speaking, heat stroke happens in the summer time, not on winter time. Frostbite happens in the wintertime, not on summer. Diarrhea or nausea often happens in the late summer as more rain come down on the late summer. As fall is a dry season, there are more symptoms related with lung; such as coughing or dry skin. Allergy in the spring is due to wind.

WIND

We don't think normally the seriousness of the wind. Let me ask you a question. You take a shower. You wash the head with shampoo. Do you open or close the mouth while the shampoo water comes down on your face? If you want to avoid the shampoo water into your mouth, you should close the mouth. But you notice by yourself that you open the mouth. If you don't realize this, try and find by yourself.

The reason is due to breathing difficulty. Then what causes this breathing difficulty? The answer is the wind. Drops of water are coming down with the air contacting. Air is also moving downward creating minor wind. Air barometric pressure falls down slightly making breathing difficulty. You may also experience the same difficult breathing during the winter time when the wind blows hard. You have to block the wind by hands at this time. This is just like old type of vaporizer. When the wind passes by fast through bottle neck, the pressure drops and the medicine come up through the straw. The wind affects our body very much.

We had swine flu from Mexico couple of years ago. Many TV stations and newspaper warn the importance of washing hands to avoid the swine flu. If no one gets swine cold, is this warning or advice effective? If anyone get sick already, this warning is alright and effective.

One man became sick with this swine flu. This man who lives in Nebraska never went to Mexico. Do you think this person didn't wash the hands and got the disease? The answer is No as this is due to the wind. Sometimes we get a warning not to go crowded places such as theater. This means we have to worry by air infection.

When swine flu was prevailed, I told patients not to worry about it. The reason is simple. As long as the body immune system is strong, the body would expel any external viruses. Another fact is that this flu began from Mexico whose temperature is high. This means wind heat based on acupuncture theory. There are number of formulas for wind heat.

DAMPNESS

We can guess that dugouts or caves are used for the living for a long time ago. There are damper in this condition than the modern houses.

This happens in this modern age, too. Some look for cheap basement rentals as the rent is expensive and this is only they can afford. As the time passes by, renters feel their body heavy.

Some suffer with edema. All happen as there are damper in the basement.

Some can tell when the rain comes, as their body such as knee pains has more dampness than normal persons. When I watch TV program, MD explains this case over barometric pressure. General audience understands the rain which is dampness, but not on barometric pressure which must be measured by the machine. How many do people be able to measure? I believe better to explain easy.

Some try to use diuretic for edema just as a reference. This may treat only symptom, but not the cause.

DRYNESS

Fall's character is dry. This season is good for harvest as the temperature falls and dampness declines.

SUMMER HEAT AND COLDNESS

This is easily understandable, so explanation is omitted.

SUGGESTION

I recommend everyone to take at least 4 times of acupuncture treatments. The reason is everyone knows seasons change every year. We can't do any things season changes, but we know that summer is hot. Why don't we make our body cooler before summer comes? Some feels cold during the treatment and asks to cover with blanket.

Fall is a dry season. Lung is connected with fall according to acupuncture theory. Lung likes dampness, but if lung becomes dry, we tend to cough or the skin becomes dry. If we get acupuncture treatments, the probability becoming dry is far less.

As winter is cold, it is better to make warm body. Spring is wind season, so get the treatment to calm down the wind.

I believe this kind of prevention is the best way to live healthy without sickness.

RESULT OF PREVENTION

There are two parts in the health insurance. One is the right to see doctors and prescription. The other is to get hospitalization. The premium of the health insurance is $12000 a year. If the cost of two parts is the same, you may expect the following result. Nobody knows when the accident happens. So we just buy this portion. However if we are healthy, we may not need the health examination and prescription drugs. So we don't buy this portion. Let us assume you get four acupuncture treatments and four people in the family and the cost of acupuncture treatments is $250 per person totaling $1000 per year. As the premium of this portion is $6000

A year, this family saves $5000 per year. This method makes you healthier and save money. Is there any better way than this? In case you need western diagnose, you pay in cash. I believe this would not exceed $5000 on most cases.

INTERNAL CAUSE

We hear a lot about stress. When we suffer without specific reasons, we may say because of stress. Where does this stress come from?

Acupuncturists believe stress comes from our 7 emotions; Joy, anger, worry, thinking too much, sadness, fear, and frighten. These are related with internal diseases. Our spirit is disturbed by outside stimulus. This leads to excessive excitement or repression causing damages on body organs.

For examples many believe that being joy is good. But excessive joy may be not good.

1. We watch TV program searching people who lost a contact for a long time. One mother explains how she lost her daughter. The curtain opens and her daughter begins to walk out and shout "Mom" and fainted and collapsed. What happened? It is because of excessive joy.

2. One person watches TV program for his Lotto. One number is the same, and second one is the same . . . . The heart starts beating harder and harder. Finally the last number is the same and the person becomes fainted

organs	Liver	Heart	Spleen	Lung	Kidney
emotion	Anger	Joy	Anxiety	Sorrow	fear

CASE 1

The variation of emotion is different with people. Some person has a tendency of leaning on one side.

This patient had a stomach cancer surgery. She was alright for the first 3 months after the surgery. Since then she had the same uncomfortable feeling just like as before the surgery. While I explained about emotions specially on thinking too much, she said "Yes, I do think too much and have anxiety always." As you see the above table, spleen and stomach are affected by anxiety and thinking too much. Her case is the original cause was the emotional matter and the symptom was shown on stomach. Her case of the surgery was done only on symptom, not on the real cause. Another interesting is person with lots of anxiety has less appetite and loose bowel movement. All these happen as spleen function is weak.

Case 2

Many people work on occupations that they can't be angry. A customer is a king, isn't it? They have to serve these customers, on any conditions. Some customers are very unreasonable and demanding to employees making stressful. Some bosses make their subordinator very nervous and stressful. Most of them can't express their emotions or protest. On many cases these would develop to depression or a disease caused by pent-up rage.

Bible says on Ephesians 4:26 "Be angry and do not sin; do not let the sun go down on your wrath."

We need some wisdom. No matter how angry we are, we must train ourselves to get out the anger before we go to bed. I personally go to the park or beach and shout it out.

3. Most cases

One emotion has a tendency to affect to all emotions. For example someone get a layoff notice. Why me? The right next guy doesn't work hard at all and get any notice at all. This fact makes angrier than his layoff. When the time passes by, it is not easy to find a new job. I have only one month of saving. If I don't find a job, he can't pay the rent making worry. He thinks hard and harder. He is afraid of being evicted and going into shelter. All these emotions may damage all organs and ultimately against the heart.

Hereditary

If someone inherited with weak organ, this may affect against emotions. For example if the person was born with weak spleen, he may have thinking more than normal. If the weak liver, he may be easily angry. It is not lucky to born with weak organs. On the top of that he becomes weaker due to this emotion. This is a vicious spiral.

If person understands all these cycles, it is required to control emotions by everyday practice. Another way is to make the weak organs strong, then emotions may affect less to organs.

THE THIRD CAUSE

There is the cause that doesn't belong to external or internal cause.

1. Damage by foods

These include unclean foods, spoiled foods, or eating too much and drinking too much.

2. Excessive labor or idleness

Sinews and bones, Qi and blood, and muscles may be damaged by excessive labor or physical idleness. You may understand easily the damage due to excessive labor. You may wonder why the physical idleness causes the damage. This means Qi becomes stagnated causing blood stagnation.

3. Sexual intemperance

Too much sexual activity will lead to the body damage due to loss of essence. We inherit the original energy from parents upon getting born. We have to keep this energy well not to lose it. This can be done by proper foods and exercises. We may use some essence if the essence is more than required. However sexual intemperance with unreasonableness will damage the body.

EXTERNAL WOUND

This means insect stung, animal biting, and cut by knife etc. This includes bruises by accidents or amputation.

4. ENVIRONMENTAL CAUSE

When buses pass by and exhausts toxic gases, it is unavoidable not to breathe the toxic air. This includes all chemical's smell.

5. EVIL QI

These are germs, bacteria and virus. Old saints guess there is something bad about germs. As they don't have microscope at that time, it is impossible to see germs by the means of enlargement. They name Evil Qi which affects bad influence to the body.

As we understand where the disease comes from, we may be easy to select which doctors we can go.

External and internal causes are better to see acupuncturists and the third cause are to see western doctors. For example the wound of disinfections and bone fracture require a surgery by western doctors.

Old acupuncture needles include surgical knives, too. Old historical novel mentioned that Hwatah did a surgery on Kwanwoo. Kwanwoo was hit by the poison arrow. While Kwanwoo played baduk with Maryang, Hwatah used mabisan as anesthesia on his arm, but not handed down unfortunately. Another story was that Hwatah asked Jojo to open his head to remove his headache. Jojo believed Hwatah may try to kill him, so Jojo killed Hwatah. One thing I want to note here is acupuncture is very effective for headache. This means acupuncture skills are improved very much compared with 1000 years ago.

However Confucianism develops and no more surgery is allowed since then. Most surgeries are done by medical doctors these days. However China has used acupuncture for anesthesia during a surgery. Patients can listen and hear in consciousness during the surgery, even the heart surgery. The cost is only one third compared with anesthesia and patients also recover faster than the regular surgery without side effects of anesthesia medicine.

Modern science did a great role about evil Qi. It is possible to observe penicillium by microscope and make antibiotics and save lots of people. Modern science also develops anatomy and makes impossible cases to be possible by the surgery. Everyone became fascinated to the new medical science. We have learned only western theories on school. For example we learned XX and XY in the biology, not on wind or damp or dry and hot & cold etc. We began to realize western science cannot answer all questions. Antibiotics and surgery can't proclaim the complete recovery, but rather make patients with chronic disease. So many people start looking for alternatives such as acupuncture.

HERE IS MY SUGGESTION.

Exterior and interior causes are well taken care of by Eastern methods and Western science can do better on the third cause.

PAINS

I go to bookstores once in a while. The fact that someone could write a book means that the author has a profound knowledge on the subject. I used to buy books on a certain field when I was young. Now I concentrate on health related issue, especially on TCM.

When I look around health sections on the book store, there is one book "As I am sick, I am young." I picked up the book and looked the content there was not a word that is related with TCM. I didn't buy the book. I heard later that book is a best seller. I learn later that it is not for physical pain, but for mental pain.

What is the cause of the pain? Very simple. It is caused by lack of oxygen and nutrition. We just believe the pain is the difficult issue, that's why it is difficult. If we think this is a simple issue, it may be simple on many cases. If oxygen and nutrition are provided into the pain area, the pain will be removed. In order to achieve this we have to remove the blockages.

There is no pain with proper blood circulation in another word on most cases. Old saints call this "Qi and blood". This is the same meaning even though the expression is different. Qi means energy. Energy means the power of moving. This power is the oxygen. Blood is the almost same meaning with western terminology. Therefore if Qi and blood go round well, there is no discomfort, pain and disease.

Therefore we try to find what the blockage is and to remove that. The story ends here. As disharmony begins with wind, cold, summer heat, damp, dry and heat, the only thing is to make the balance between them. Qi and blood get weaker in the beginning. This weakness changes into Qi and blood stagnation, blood stasis and phlegm. It is relatively easy to treat in the beginning, but if this becomes into chronicle, it becomes more difficult to treat. In the meantime patients suffer more and cost more expensive to treat.

Our body has the ability to cure by itself. We ignore this ability and depend on the idea of excessive chemical medicines and the surgery.

ALLERGY IN SPRING

Patients who suffer with allergic rhinitis are weak on their immune system and respond sensitively. Rhinitis accompany with nose running, nose stuffiness and sneezing, but also headache, chronic fatigue, less ability on concentration, tardy growth and sleeping problem etc. This causes bringing down quality of life. This rhinitis develops into empyema. Some suffer with itchy eyes, lots of tears and even form of pus on eyes.

We have learned only western side such as biology, but not on traditional oriental medicine. We never thought the fundamental reason why allergy prevails on spring. We just look at the existing state only, not the real cause. Therefore the cause remains the same.

We have learned that plants wait for animals or people to come to them for their reproduction. For example we learned that animals eat some fruits and excrete seeds nearby that are not digested. In this way plants maintain their species, but also multiply. When people or animals pass, thorn or prickle may go along with them, and then spread everywhere.

If so, how do plants multiply if they are located where people or animals are difficult to reach?

Plants know that where they are is the best place for them. Simply speaking this is the hometown. We live in the northern hemisphere. The wind blows after the spring equinox. This wind is a soft wind or gentle breeze. When this wind blows, pollens are blown away. This wind is not like strong hurricane or typhoon. As strong wind may send pollen far away, plants don't like the strong wind. This wind may break or damage plants, so plants may not like this strong wind. Pollen that is blown by the wind floats about in the air. While people breathe through the nose and mouth, pollen enters into our body and cause spring allergy.

Therefore I define the spring allergy as a symptom caused by the wind. Everyone knows there is almost no allergy while raining. The allergy is caused by the wind. The wind is by the broad meaning and pollen is by narrow meaning.

According to oriental medicine the wind is considered all causes of diseases. I believe this concept can apply not only to human being but also to animals. Foot and mouth disease of animals becomes a big issue in Korea. Government believes this disease is caused by human contact. The government tries to limit access from people of out of town. They try to disinfect all cars in and out of town. But this disease spread fast to neighbor towns. One news report spreading is caused by the epidemic preventer. In the meantime there is news that North Korea has the same problem. Does South Korean epidemic preventer go to North Korea? All these happen as they don't consider this disease spread by the wind.

Another reason may be as cows grow in the narrow barn instead of raising cattle in the wide pasture, cattle can't do necessary exercise causing their immune system weaker.

This disease usually goes away when spring comes. This means this germ has more heat in itself. When the temperature is low, this germ can survive, but not on warm temperature. We can conclude this germ belongs to wind heat in the terminology of oriental medicine. We may use the same principle to find the cause of allergy in the same way.

How can we treat spring allergy? There are two methods for general publics. The first is to take honey. Who makes honey? The answer is bees. Bees don't care about pollen. Pollen doesn't do anything against bees. These bees make honey. Therefore if you take honey for a long time, your body may improve against pollen. Please note that all honeys are not equal. You have to take honey which is produced within a radius of one hour driving that is 50-60 miles. Someone who lives in New York should not take cactus honey which is produced in Arizona. The factor or gene for allergy is from where I live.

The second is buying pollen from local bee yard. Take pollen with one spoon a day. You feel the difference within a month. This is the same concept that poison can be treated by a poison.

When you have itchy eyes, try to wash with cold water, but don't rub eyes. If you rub eyes, it will make worse. Or you can put your head into the refrigerator toward where cold air blows. If you experience itchy throat, try to have ice cream. Itchy throat means heat in the throat. Drive a car with the window closed. Turn A/C instead. This will avoid pollen while driving.

Try to avoid going out in the morning as this wind is stronger during morning time. Morning time belongs to liver based on acupuncture theory. Try to use A/C in the house instead of opening windows.

Our body has immunity system to take care of exterior cause. There are two groups of people on the same condition of spring allergy. Some suffer so much and others don't understand why some people suffer because of allergy. People who suffer have weak immune system in other words. Acupuncturists explain this condition "deficiency". Do you think any other reasons?

Let me explain more details. Running nose means spleen function is weak. Sneezing means weak lung. Itchy throat means due to heat. The organ to take care of heat is ultimately kidney, so itchy throat means weak kidney function. However spring belongs to liver, so allergy comes from weak liver function in the end.

Acupuncture treatment is the number one consideration and works well. Most patients experience runny nose becomes dry while needles are on. The second is to tonify the immune system using oriental herbs.

1. Some patients use anti histamine or anti biotic. When the symptom is weak, these medicines help. However long term uses makes immune system weak, but also damages the stomach. Some suffer with stomach ulcer on the worst case.

2. Some get a shot. I understand most shots are steroid. The problem is liver try to detoxify steroid and kidney to excrete. Steroid is the double edged sword. It is all right that condition improves with a little use. Over or long term use may cause liver function, kidney function and bones weak. This may result immune system further weaker.

3. Some try protective inoculations for weeks and years on worst cases. Who has the insurance must pay a copayment each time every week. Depending on conditions, some take once for the first 3 months and once every two weeks afterward and gradually less.

    Allergy may still continue with long period of treatment on some cases. An antibody is made against the original gene, Upon the new test, the body need another antibody, and new treatments require. All these mean allergy comes from low immune system. Therefore the best way is to strengthen the immune system to avoid spring allergy every year.

4. I suggest practicing this acupressure. Press hegu with other thumb which is located in the middle between thumb and index finger.

    Second spot is quchi. When the elbow is flexed, this spot is in the depression at the internal end of the transverse cubital crease.

    Please note when you use too often and the effectiveness will be reduced, it is better off randomly.

WHY DON'T WE EAT FRESHWATER FISH AS SLICED RAW FISH?

The principal of yin and yang applies to all natures. Sliced raw fish is from sea fishes. All creatures try something not to be rotten or spoiled. Most popular method is using sea salt. There is the least amount of salt in the water of a brook and are plenty in the sea. Freshwater fishes try to hold salt in their body to prevent rottening. In the other hand sea fish try to push out salt as they are surrounded by sea salt. Therefore sea fishes are rather unsaline but dainty, and freshwater fishes taste salty. Fishes with thick flesh like mackerel need more seasoning with salt. Freshwater fishes are good for pepper pot soup or hot chowder. All fishes know how to survive in the nature. Gathering and pushing out is a part of yin and yang.

Trees look dead in the winter. New buds and green leaves begin to grow in the spring. Trees try to pull salt in the air through new buds. The unbalance occurs in the tree. Upper part has more salt and lower part has less salt. The trees try hard to push up water through roots to make a balance. This is the osmosis in physics. This is another type of survival.

When we breathe, a tiny amount of salt in the air enters into the body. We may say this happens more in the beach area. However we may guess less salt in the body as trees and plants use more. Therefore it is desirable to consume a little extra salt in the spring.

Have you put a piece of slide of potato on skin burn? Why? As potato has cold nature and fire is hot nature, this combination makes a balance each other. Potato has a tendency to grow on the surface of the earth. Potatoes try to get more sunshine.

What about cucumber? Cucumbers grow well with a rod standing up. Cucumbers try to grow up towards the sun. This means cucumbers belong to cold food. Radish grows downward under the ground. Radishes try to run away from the sun instead of approaching to the sun. Therefore radish has warm nature. What about ginseng that everyone knows? When you look at roots, there are not any roots toward the sky rather into the ground. Therefore ginseng is the herb that makes body warm. Without knowing this kind of nature, what is going to happen if warm person takes ginseng? If so, warm body becomes warmer, this is not desirable.

Let us consider about mushroom. Mushrooms always grow at shades. Shades are cool and sunny spots are warm. Why do mushrooms grow at only at shades? The answer is its personality is hot. If mushrooms grow at sunny spots, they are going to burn. That's why they want to grow at shades. If cold person takes mushrooms, the body becomes warm and it is good for the body. However mushrooms may be harmful for warm person. If warm person takes them as they believe mushrooms may prevent cancer, do you think this prevents cancer? I have seen many who doesn't know the cancer condition and take mushrooms.

Let us consider cactus. Cactus is used a lot for constipation. Many use cactus without considering patient's condition. One of the reasons for constipation is due to heat. Cactus usually grows at the desert. The desert is hot and dry. In order to survive on desert condition, any plants that can live must have opposite character; cold and wet. Therefore cactus is cold and wet in nature.

If heat resides on the large intestine, there is less damp. In this case cactus is very good on heat type of constipation. Cold and wet damp make a balance against heat and dry of constipation making yin and yang in balance. What about the constipation caused by cold? Do you think cactus is going to work? Unless you understand well, the condition may be worse. Therefore we can conclude it may be dangerous on using something for everything.

As you can understand now, all plants or foods have different types of energy (Qi). Therefore it is desirable to take foods depending on personal constitution.

Foods are the foundation of health

Let me ask a question. Why is cola bad for the health? Most answer that cola contains sugar and caffeine, that's why it is not good. Some says it is made by carbonic acid and this acid has a tendency of dissolving bones. For example, put a tooth taken out from the child mouth into cola. The tooth becomes like marshmallow. However there is no one who holds cola for 2 or 3 days in the mouth, so this is the only a theory and not practical. However drinking cola for a long time could affect teeth in the long run.

We learned in the primary school that when we breathe in, oxygen enters into the body and we breathe out carbon dioxide comes out of the body. Oxygen combines with nutrition and supplies oxygen and nutrition into body cells. Through this process oxygen changes into carbon dioxide. So we may say oxygen is good for the body and carbon dioxide is bad for the body.

What is the carbonated water? Adding carbon dioxide into water is carbonated water. When we drink cola, some of the gas comes out by burping and the rest of gas goes into the body. All gas must be absorbed by our cells. All cells have to work hard to get rid of carbonic dioxide. Do we have to buy expensive drinks and make our body work hard unnecessarily?

Cola may be good for indigestion especially food stagnation. This is the reason cola becomes popular. One client asked for indigestion. The clerk mixed a few things and gave to the client. The client came back and asked the same thing again as the taste was so good and it helped for indigestion. This is the beginning of the famous Coca Cola.

However if anyone suffers with food stagnation, it is better off to take care of the root cause rather drinking cola. The function of stomach is to receive foods from the mouth and make foods into porridge type which is easy to absorb and send to the small intestine. The small intestine is located under the stomach. The energy of the stomach is supposed to downward. This is normal. If the stomach energy is upward such as frequent burping or even vomiting, this means abnormal.

When I was in master degree of oriental medine, a professor of nutritional science supplied some interesting column. One Indian who was born in Alaska used to catch and eat salmons, whales and even bears when he was young. When he grew up, he became a nutritionist and recommended his clients to eat more vegetables and he also eats more vegetables by himself. Unfortunately he became sick and was hospitalized. He gave a thought why he became sick, even though he just followed by the book. He recalled he was healthy and strong when he was young. He tried to eat some meats before he dies. He became healthy and strong after he started to eat meats. Some claims that eating only vegetables may be harmful from this story. Some vegetarians conclude this is a rare and special case.

However if you interpret this with yin and yang, it is so simple. We know Alaska is the place generally cold. This person was born in cold place meaning he has more yin energy, which is cold. It is the basic principle to make the balance between yin and yang. With this principle this person must take more in warm foods. Salmons, whales and bears belong to yang and warm nature. For example polar bears play on ice and snow. This is possible as bears have warm body. However most vegetables belong to the yin meaning cool or cold. The yin person takes yin foods causing sick so take yang foods making healthy.

We can't explain the above story with carbohydrate, protein, fat, vitamin and mineral. This is the western approach. For example zinc is good for prostate issue. Zinc is included in oyster and pumpkin seed. However this approach can't be explained by oriental medicine.

In the other hand oriental medicine classifies by the taste such as sour, bitter, sweet, spicy and salty. This is the oriental approach by the tastes. We can understand we must take all tastes to become healthy. If we choose tastes only what we like, we would become sick. Most of us don't like bitter taste. Some oriental herbs taste bitter. In Korea there is a proverb "medicine has bitter taste".

What did old ancients do without microscopes? Carbohydrate, protein and fat eventually change into glucose, so sweet taste. Sour taste may be vitamin C as lemon containing with vitamin C is sour. Salty taste may be sodium. What about spicy taste according to western classification? What about the bitter taste?

There is no perfect one in theory. Western theory has its own merit and eastern medicine also has its own merit. The combination of two systems may make better alternatives to general public for healthy foods.

Please note that all vegetables don't belong to yin and all animals belong to yang. There is no absolute in acupuncture theory. It is just like a magnet. The magnet point's one side is north and the other side is south. Let us cut this magnet exactly in half. It is supposed to be neutral, but the fact is each ends again point south and north. Yin and yang is just like a magnet. Yin and yang in the health is to fulfill the insufficiency. Let us think about how to use yin and yang theory into the selection of foods.

Why is not good as a food on white flour and rice?

When I was in Korea in young age, I used to eat rice. Since I came to USA, I often had toast instead of rice in the morning. The bread has a level "enriched". Have you seen the level "enriched"? The bread made of whole wheat doesn't have the word of enriched in written. White flour is cut off the shell which contains vital nutrient. Many consumers complain about the lack of nutrients from the white bread. Bread companies add chemical nutrients instead of natural ones.

In order to explain the reason why white flour products are not good for healthy, let me think about how to make a paste. When I was young, we use wallpapers for decorating the wall. We cover the paste behind wallpaper and attach to the wall. When I was a kid, my parent put the white flour into the bin and adds water. They stirred the bin once in a while not to make burn. Over the time white flour changes into a sticky paste. This is the process of creating a paste.

The foods with white flour mix with water, broth or soda in the stomach. When the stomach receives the above food, the stomach tries to digest food and secretes gastric juice and start peristalsis. The stomach is supposed to be warm or hot. This process is very identical just like making the paste: the combination of white flour, water and heat. These foods have changed like paste and sent to the small intestine through the pyloric. The small intestine is supposed to absorb all nutrients. The small intestine is consisted with villi that are able to maximize the surface area to absorb the nutrients. If the paste covers the villi, the paste prevents absorbing the nutrients through the villi. All good nutrients will be excreted. When this condition continues, the belly will appear.

The products of shells cut off are sold for treating constipation at high prices. Some understand this kind of the fact and some don't. However they still stick to white flour bread or products. The reason is simple. The taste is better. Whole wheat products are usually harsh and the taste is less.

White flour and white rice are preferred by the same reason. North Korea's leader Kim Il Sung called his goal to feed white rice and meat broth for the people in North Korea. In South Korea some take boiled rice and cereals instead of white rice. The preference of brown rice is far less. One of the reasons is tough to eat. I tell you how to eat brown rice that contain the original nutrients and eliminate drawbacks.

Rice belongs to Earth in acupuncture theory. Earth is the foundation of all things. Rice is well balanced with others, wood, earth, fire, metal and water. Make fire with wood. Metal or stone rice bowl contains water with rice. So we can say rice is the food well balanced in yin and yang.

Brown rice is very helpful as it contains lots of fiber. When eating outside personally on some occasions, I don't have much choice or forced to eat the white flour products. Eating very little white flour foods is better than to starve. I weigh next day and find I gain two pounds, even though I ate a little white flour foods. There is almost no difference between a lot or less in white flour foods.

As I don't eat white flour foods, my wife doesn't cook them often. My wife could not believe this fact in the beginning. She realized and experienced the same thing in gaining weight. Do you want to lose weight? Eat brown rice from now on.

First, put brown rice and white rice separately in water and wait for a few days. Brown rice sprouts, but white rice doesn't do, rather the body start to disappear. In other word, brown rice has life force and white rice has no vitality. As our each body cells have vitality, don't you agree to take the brown rice that provides vitality?

Where vitamins and minerals are made, brown rice is geminated on purpose. The reason is this process increase the amount of vitamins and minerals. If germinated brown rice is taken at home, it is much easier to eat as plain brown rice force us lots of chewing and cause the pain on jaw joint. However the germination reduces this burden less.

Soak the brown rice in water. Changing the water needs in the morning and evening. If not changed, the water smells rotten. In the winter it may take a week depending on room temperature. But it takes just one day in the summer. While changing the water, take a closer look whether buds come out. One important thing is the buds should be 0.2-0.5mm. If the buds are too large, nutrients will be reduced by using buds grow too much. If you still have rice left on the rice cooker, keep germinated rice into the refrigerator to prevent further grow. There are rice cooker on the market that is able to germinate, so this is other option. There also is germinated brown rice on the market, too.

Many people tell since they eat the brown rice and their body has improved. According to four types of constitution, brown rice doesn't console for Tai yang, but I don't agree personally. Maybe I am wrong, so I suggest trying for the 3 months. If any abnormal symptom shows, you may discontinue.

WHAT IS YIN AND YANG?

I guess that old sages came up with the concept of yin and yang by the long experience. Day comes when the night passes and one day passes. This process is repeated. Then seasons are changed; spring, summer, autumn and winter making one year. This is repeated endlessly. The sun rise in the morning and the moon rises at the night. This is also repeated. What does this have an orderly manner in place? They concluded all things begin from yin and yang.

In the East they did not know God's existence what the Bible describes. I think how wise old sages were and they found the existence of yin and yang based on experience and thought and philosophy. Let me compare with the Bible as many people believe in the Bible and go to church.

Yin and yang is the opposite concept, but exists together.

Let us look at Genesis Chapter5 verses 3 to 5.

Then God said "Let there be the light." And there was light. And God saw the light that it was good and God divided the light from the darkness. He called Night. So the evening and the morning were the first day.

Light and darkness is just yin and yang. Light and darkness that we understand today is from the light of sun and moon and stars created on the fourth day. These lights are different from what is created on the first day. In my opinion, if we use the concept of yin and yang of the first day, the interpretation of Bible is a little easier about the light on the first day.

Another thing I notice is the darkness may be already existed inside of the light or before the light the darkness already existed.

That's why God divided the light from the darkness. In another word, yin and yang exists together.

Another example is that yin and yang is just like a magnet. One side points to the south and the other side points to the north. Cut the exact center. Theoretically the center must be a neutral. But neither pieces the south nor the north. Each piece shows north and south again contrary to the theory.

From the above Bible, there are two examples in yin and yang. The first is light and darkness. The second is morning and evening. If you look at the genesis based on yin and yang, we can divide into heaven and earth, earth and sea, great light (sun) and lesser light (moon) and animals and vegetables . . .

Examples

Day and night, cold and hot, past and future, expansion and contraction, up and down, life and death, good and bad, inhale and exhale, mind and body, forward and backward, mass and energy, progressive and conservative, desire and ablation, deduce and inductive, man and woman, love and hate, smooth and rigidity, plus and subtraction, multiplication and division, and there are endless.

Let us think about for a moment to view for the softness and firmness. I told you already that there is no absolute in yin and yang and these two always exist together. The man has the softness inside and the rigidity outside. On the other hand the woman has the softness outside and the rigidity inside.

When woman is young, as the softness exists outside, she is sweet, cute, friendly and charming. Man shows bluntly and valiant as the hardness is outside. When man and woman marry, it may interpret hardness and softness combines. Theoretically rigidity overwhelms softness meaning man may win over woman in the beginning. However as the time pass by, the boss at work makes hard, his subordinators drive up crazy and customers always demand as a king. Gradually all hardness disappear making man packed with the softness outside. Man is educated not to show tears, so the softness remains inside. However man starts to cry, he bursts into tears more severely than girls cry as the softness resides inside. On the other hand woman exhausts all softness in order to survive in the wild world and only the rigidity left over. As time passes married woman's voice is stronger and this is the principal of yin and yang.

When woman becomes a widow, there is a tendency she does everything for taking care of her children at all costs. Mom works hard until all rigidity wear out. So that's why we call Mom great.

Look at mushrooms. While growing in the soil, it is so soft. Once it becomes dry, it becomes so hard. This is the reason that original nature of mushroom is hard. Squid is also true. While squid is alive, it is tender feeling, but when it dries in the fire, it becomes very hardened. This is because the original nature of squid is hard.

Ladies and gentlemen, more you understand yin and yang; it becomes easier and also interesting. Before I study TCM (traditional Chinese medicine) and yin and yang, I thought yin and yang as superstition existed in the past or treat it as one old system at best. When I study more and more, I go deeply into the depth of old ancient's wisdom.

If yin and yang in genesis of Bible is the universe, yin and yang of TCM belongs to microcosm. The sky means head, 4 directions of north, south, east and west means extremities of arms and legs. Airflow means energy, lightening; anger, dew; sweat, wind; dizziness, and 5 continent 6 ocean; 5 zhang 6 fu. Water occupy 75% of the earth and 75% of the body is also water. 5 elements theory is the foundation of operation of microcosm. The next subject is 5 elements theory.

One of the classic of the classics says that yin and yang is the way of heaven and earth. It is the law that controls everything. This is the main subject that causes the change of raising and killing. It is where the spirit resides. All diseases must be healed by adjusting yin and yang.

This means if you don't know yin and yang, you can't treat the diseases.

What are 5 elements?

Western Philosophy

In the West, especially in Greece, they thought that the world consists of four kinds of material. They are air, fire, earth, and water. I have learned this in collage 46 years ago. This is combined with each other and creates hot, cold, wet and dry. This also creates spring, summer, autumn and winter. If you apply this into human beings, these are heart, liver, spleen and brain.

Eastern philosophy

The universe is composed of five substances; wood, fire, earth, metal and water. This is the basis of the five elements. This notion began based on birth, growth, harvest and conceal. This is the order of the universe so to speak. The buds grow into the ground and become abundant in growth and leaves and flowers and branches etc. This will result in fruits and seeds. Seeds fall and hide to the ground. And these rotations continue. Everything that control is based on earth or soil.

The original meaning of the oriental medicine is a little more difficult for general public to understand, so I try to explain easily to understand. There are two different cycles. One is a promotional cycle and the other is an antagonistic cycle. The promotional one is helping each other. This can be the concept of parent and child. This means mother does the best and accepts for the child. In the contrast when the child becomes better, the parent feels elated and has rewarding feeling.

On the other hand, if parents love the child without conditions or restrictions, the child may be spoiled and rude. Therefore we need someone who is strict and deters rude behavior. We call this as a father. This is the law of the jungle. The strong one harasses the weak one.

PROMOTIONAL CYCLE

Wood means tree. Fire can be burn well with wood. Without wood fire is extinguished. Dust left over after fire extinguished. Minerals are in the soil and dust. Minerals can hold flowing water. You can guess that good water comes out of rocks containing lots of minerals. You can also think reservoirs hold water. Water can make tree grow. Trees can't grow without water. We call this relationship as a promotional cycle. We also call these; wood creates fire, fire creates soil, soil creates metal, metal creates water and water creates tree.

ANTAGONISTIC CYCLES

As trees are rooted in the soil, trees bother the dirt. The soil can block water. Think of a dam. The water can shut off the fire. The fire can change the form of metal. Think of the furnace. Knifes or saws made by iron can cut down the tree. When you read or study oriental medicine, you may sometimes encounter mutual or antagonistic cycles. If you remember this information, this would be helpful to understand better.

5 ELEMENTS AND HUMAN BODY

Wood	Fire	Earth	Metal	Water
Liver	Heart	Spleen	Lung	Kidney
Gallbladder	Small intestine	Stomach	Large intestine	Urinary bladder
Eye	Tongue	Mouth	Nose	Ear
Spring	Summer	Late summer	Autumn	Winter
Sour	Bitter	Sweet	Spicy	Salty
Anger	Joy	Think	Sorrow	Fear
Tendon	Blood	Flash	Skin	Bone
Tear	Sweat	Saliva	Mucous	Urine
Nails	Complexion	Lips	Body hair	Head hair
Wind	Hot	Damp	Dryness	Cold
Green/blue	Red	Yellow	White	Black

This table is important to diagnose. For example if a lot of tears come out, we know the liver may be associated. The person who is angry easier may be due to the liver function. Red face means heart problem. Please try to recall President Clinton. Everyone knows he had a heart surgery. However I knew he had a heart problem before his surgery. While he served as a president, he had a sex scandal. He protested with pointing fingers that he didn't have with her on TV. His face was red at the time. His face looks normal on TV these days. This means his heart condition improved. This simple idea may predict health problem far earlier than most medical tests.

CONCLUSION

The 5 element helps each other, but often restraints on the other hand. The balance will be maintained in this way. Antagonistic cycle is similar with Murphy's Law and promotional cycle is with Sally' law. This means one organ becomes bad, and then another organ will follow. You know the Domino game. One card built falls with the touch of the first card and hits another in a row and continues to the end. However we do not need to be disappointed as one organ becomes better and then another organ becomes better. Therefore five elements are important as all treatments begin with five elements.

We live in this world that cannot escape from Yin and yang. Even Goku can fly into the sky, we shouldn't forget he played only in the palm of the Buddha. Believe it or not we always live in yin and yang with 5 elements. For example look at the calendar. Sunday and Monday represent yin and yang meaning sun and moon. Tuesday, Wednesday, Thursday, Friday and Saturday are 5 stars in the sky meaning Mars, Mercury, Jupiter, Venus and Saturn that are 5 elements.

CONCRETE DESCRIPTION OF YIN AND YANG AND 5 ELEMENTS

There was a King in China who was good in politics. Now and then whoever makes his people well by providing enough foods is the best king. In other words nowadays the economy is the most important subject. At the time planting well at the farms was very necessary for expecting good harvests. This is a short cut. They found that day comes by night and night comes by day. They also became aware that one season has changed to another season over time. But they found that this is constantly repeated by experience. Old ancients gradually realized that this is associated with the sky, sun and moon. The king made astronomers observe. Some observed the east and the south and others observed the west and the north. According to their observation there were a route of the sun and the moon. There were 28 nonmoving stars and 7 moving stars. They found seven moving stars impact very significantly on agriculture. They also found that the four seasons occur along the movement of the seven moving stars. These are spring, summer, autumn and winter. The calendar that we use is based on seven stars.

One old lyric of popular songs says "Persian prince who does the divination by the stars". I may guess this prince may be one of the three wise men. Whether my guess is right or not, this nation used the calendar with one week. The calendar we use currently also is being used one week as a unit. There is no distinction between the east and the west. Old people didn't know the Bible, but they found the number seven by observing the order of heaven. The Bible said God made the heaven and the earth in a week. Do you think this is a coincidence?

Our calendar begins with Sunday and Monday and ends on Saturday. Most do not know what this means even though we use in everyday life. Sunday represents the sun and Monday represents the moon meaning yin and yang. From Tuesday to Saturday represents Mars, Mercury, Jupiter, Venus and Saturn in the sky. There are 5 elements in the earth and 5 stars in the sky.

Healthy life style-
Good bowel movement

People say that if you have good sleeping, eating and bowel movement, people cannot be ill. This is easy to say, but keeping this is not that easy. There are so many people who suffer from insomnia. Some young person suffering with insomnia often begins to sleep on the table as soon as needles are inserted, but the older patients are not that easy.

Meaning of Good Bowel Movement

Let me tell you the story easy. In the medical field it defines who goes to bowel movement once every 2 days at least is not on constipation. I am against this theory. I believe that stool at least daily is considered normal. When we eat foods, the mouth chews up and sends down foods to the stomach through the esophagus. The food becomes the dough in the stomach. The action of the stomach is that upper wall pushes down and lower wall lifts to make foods into the dough. This movement takes 3-5 hours depending on foods. Foods send down further through pyloric into the duodenum where digestive juices come from gallbladder and pancreas. Small intestine absorbs all the nutrition and the remaining residue sends to the large intestine. The colon serves to absorb the necessary moisture. It takes 12 hours from the mouth to the rectum.

There is a circadian clock which shows the weak or active time of organs. The time of the large intestine is between 5:00 and 7:00 in the morning. This means the most appropriate time for the bowel movement to the rhythm of the body. Most people wake up in the morning and go to the bathroom with the newspaper. This is just due to the usual body rhythm.

So we eat breakfast and lunch. However it is important what time is for the dinner. Of course the time for the breakfast is important, but now we talk about the bowel movement. Let us assume that you have the dinner between 6:00 and 6:30 in the evening. After 12 hours later all foods you ate are ready to come out. If any left over from yesterday comes out, it can define as good bowel movement.

If you eat the dinner at 9:00 in the evening, this food is not ready yet for the bowel movement and fails to come out. Person must wait until the next morning. Do you have any good reason to keep this smelly stool until the next day?

There is another reason for the late dinner. The late dinner will interfere with other organs operation. For example if the meal is taken at 9:00 pm, all bloods supposed to move into triple burner can't gather at the right time and spot. Triple burner will be weakening by the repeated action. Now you may understand how important your regular meal time is.

CONSTIPATION

Even though you go to the bathroom for the urge, nothing comes out or difficult. Nothing comes out no matter trying to push hard. Some patients wear plastic glove after applying Vaseline on the finger and stick into the rectum and take out feces. Why does this happen?

1. The moving form of intestine is called peristalsis. It is just like a snake's winding movement. If there is lack of peristalsis movement, it is likely causing the constipation. Eating high fiber diet is recommended by MD. TCM classifies the cause; Qi deficiency, cold colon or heat colon. Some older people who are incapacitated in the bed all day have a tendency of the constipation. It is due to Qi deficiency. Walking fast is recommended. A better way is to jump a rope.

When your body moves up and down, the large intestine also moves up and down helping peristaltic movement automatically.

2. I already mentioned that the large intestine absorbs water. For some reason, the body especially in the large intestine becomes warmer. This will cause the colon absorbs more moisture. If there is less water in the stool, the stool becomes stiffer. Many recommend drinking more water, but the effect is negligible. If you drink plenty of water, this only increase a lot of urine instead of helping with the constipation. The reason is that the small intestine separates the water and sends water into the urinary bladder. This is the oriental theory.

CONCLUSION

We need to know which causes the constipation. There are lots of reasons; eating too little, less body fluid, damp heat etc. There are lots of side effects that general people don't understand; such as acne, freckles and even rough skin. Even though you understand the cause, there is a case that patients cannot move. We recommend acupuncture treatments. It requires one to three treatments. We also recommend a drinking tea depending on patient's condition.

Why do we use only white mouse in the laboratory?

White dressed people test white mouse for the test. My question is why only white mouse are used, even though most mouse are black or brown. Black or brown mice look fast and white mice look slow. I have never seen white mice in typical home or field. That's why I don't understand the reason to use or test with white mouse. The validity of the statistics law is from more objects with the highest number, but this law is not applicable on this case. I wonder why and search the internet. The following comes from the internet.

"White mouse are suited the best as more effect with less expenses. Experimental results must appear well, easy to manage genetically, easy to manage with low cost, short generation, possible for mass rearing, easy carcass processing, and meets many appropriate parts with human beings.

Therefore we create mice with mutations and breed white mice. White mice are special species by mutation for the experimental purposes. White mice look less disgusting and we can see the result easily. So we can say these are economical, easy to manage and fast to get the desired results and white mice are best suited for."

There were many good reasons of course, but not listed here for all. The description makes a sense on some points, but this doesn't explain everything to me. I understand the lab must be clean, so white color may be number one color to be clean. Western tradition continued the same way everywhere even in Korea. The only difference is a yellow person.

White person wearing white gown tests with white mouse. Why is everything white? I mentioned there are 5 different colors in the oriental system. If this applies to people, there are Mongoloid Asians, westerners Caucasian, and African black. I assume Avatar in the movie may belong to Green. There are not only different skin color, but also different hair color; black, yellow, and red (4% of the world's population). One thing in common is as we get older, the hair color changes into white. Hair shape is also different. In particular most blacks have curly hair. Eye color is different. There are black, blue and yellow colors of eyes. Do you think all people have the same size of organs? I think the strength of organs may vary and be different depending on the races.

For example, when we go to the dermatologist, MD manages your skin with a laser. Interesting fact is more effective for the white and yellow and black results less effective. The reason is the laser was created for whites. The skin of whites ages faster than other races. They look older than other races compared even though in the same age group. The skin belongs to lung and white color belongs to lung. I hope this makes some sense to you.

Therefore this is my opinion that testing white mouse focus predominantly on the white even though the original purpose was not intended in this way. No matter what, is it true that the color of mouse is white? When we use different color mouse like brown for the same symptoms, the result may be slightly different in my opinion. If the test is on brown or black mouse, better drug family may come out for the yellow and the black. However I am doubtful that investors who want to maximize profits would accept this proposal.

Penicillin is made of blue mold. Blue mold grows where the dampness prevails. I don't know all the details how blue mold fungus develop and change, however the fundamental properties like the dampness. If you use these drugs to people whose body contains more dampness, these drugs may have side effects to them. Even though the person didn't have any side effects in the past, penicillin may show side effects if the person has damp at this moment. We must read and be aware of this fact making possible to cope in the emergency. When I visit doctor's office, there is a question and answer in personal information about being allergic to penicillin. This question means that penicillin can cause side effects. Of course I am aware that when penicillin was created, a test was done to a person instead of rats.

In the laboratory we assume all people in the world are the same. But Mr. Lee Jaema in Korea claimed that different drug should be used based on different constitution. This theory was conceived in the study where the area of Korea is relatively small and modest compared with other territory. But do you think the world be like? I believe that the concept of constitution is a freaky idea. He used same prescription per person against similar symptoms, and discovered some people heal better and some don't. He must be a pioneer in this field of logic. Prescription drugs will be needed to do in this way. Good medicine means to take into consideration of the patient's constitution as well rather than just symptoms. However I prefer to divide five groups instead of four groups. This will be explained later.

The food does the same thing. Eating for self-constitution is the basic of the foundation of good health.

Diabetes Treatment

Is this possible to cure diabetes by oriental medicine?

There was no tool for measuring diabetes in the old days. So how would they know diabetes?

The first thing is to go out to pee. If ants gather in urine, this may show diabetes. People in old days use the habits that ants like sweet things.

The second thing is to check the underwear. As we get older, we have a tendency of pissing a little bit unto the underwear. If there is a lot of sugar in the urine, the urine turns stiff as drying.

The third thing is to check the remains of the pot. Collect the urine into the pot and boil it until all urine is evaporated. Taste the remains by finger tips. If the taste is sweet, this is diabetes.

Who can say this is not scientific? In the old books different terminology is used instead of diabetes. This follows three kinds of symptoms; polydipsia, polyuria and polyphagia. It is natural if we drink plenty of water, we piss a lot. Another real issue is over polyphagia. This means abnormal heat stays at the stomach causing fast digestion. This heat also explains drinking more water in order to eliminate the heat.

In the beginning of the diabetes it may be simple to treat as we just eliminate the heat. The problem is many people pass this time without knowing this stage. This can be prevented in advance by visiting acupuncture clinics on regular basis of four times a year. Most of people don't come to clinics for various reasons and find it too late on many cases. Then you get the advice about the diabetes which is a lifelong friend.

The worst thing is if you do not manage well, you will suffer from various complications. What should we do if we didn't discover in a timely manner? In old books, if you take certain medication for a long time, diabetes is removed permanently. This means successful therapeutic experience in the past.

In modern medicine there are two types of diabetes; type 1 and type 2 by explanation of insulin. Patients know more information better than I know. This means so many suffer with diabetes nowadays. Modern medicines ask to take diabetes medicine and encourage exercising more. I read the newspaper the other day the king asked his fat son to walk always according to the part of the Annals. Ancients don't know the insulin, but they know the exercise is good for diabetes. It is common that exercise is good. It doesn't matter even from East or West. No matter how busy noblemen are, they were not supposed to run. Modern medicines say that the best for diabetes is having a walk. Walking consumes more energy than running. So become a nobleman instead of vulgar.

When I check the patient pulse with diabetes sometimes, he seems to be non-diabetic. He may overtake the drugs. In the other hand I advise someone to be careful about the diabetes who has never diagnosed. They try not to believe what I said. They also said the last blood tests didn't show any diabetes a couple of months ago. This may be just started. This is a good example for an early detection and prevention.

There may be something in common with pulse condition for diabetes. For example pulse checkup shows the difference between pregnant woman and non-pregnant. Therefore my personal opinion is not to check the blood glucose level everyday using precious blood drop. What about the diagnosis by acupuncturists as they are able to detect the diabetes?

THE REASON OF BECOMING LOWER BLOOD GLUCOSE AFTER EXERCISE

Everyone advise to try exercising for diabetes. Blood glucose was higher before exercise, but after exercise the measurement again returns to normal. Why is that? So far there is no good explanation. This is just another hypothesis on my own. Insulin is supposed to enter into cells. If the size of insulin is larger than the gate of the cell, insulin is not able to get into the cell. After the exercise the heat produces. Heat has a tendency to expend. Cells swell and the gate of the cell also becomes larger than insulin, then the insulin will be able to get into the gate. If this hypothesis is right, the conclusion is that the size of insulin has been created larger than normal.

For another example blood clots come out during menstrual period. This chunk is unusually larger size and gives a lot of pain to women. As well as the abnormal larger size of the period provides a lot of pain, the abnormal insulin size from pancreas is the reason for diabetes in my opinion. This means the function of pancreas is not normal to produce the right size.

On the other hand this hypothesis does not apply if the patient always has a lot of body heat. On this case it is better to remove the body heat.

HOW TO IMPROVE

So what will improve the function of the spleen is to control the circulation of blood of coming into and going out from the pancreas. This is the most basic thing. In case of heat, I recommend taking oriental herb to eliminate damp heat. If Qi and blood are deficient, take also acupuncture treatment. When you come back to normal glucose level, exercise and diet alone may be able to control glucose level. So don't worry about diabetes. Get the oriental treatment instead. Any diabetes would company with other bad symptoms, but most symptoms will be disappeared in the course of treatments.

Ginseng and red ginseng and vegetables

Ginseng helps body weakness due to the lack of vigor, malaise, fatigue, sweating a lot. Ginseng also treats loss of appetite, vomiting, diarrhea caused by weak spleen and stomach function. This is used for shortness of breath due to weakening of lung function and for thirsty and diabetes caused by damage on body fluids. This is widely used for many uses and really good herb. I mentioned already ginseng has warm nature.

Red ginseng is made by steaming fresh ginseng and dried. In the process on steamed and dried are produced flavonoids, B vitamins, antioxidants, amino acids. These are superior to fresh ginseng for strengthening immune system and blood circulation, inhibiting the formation of blood clots and anti-aging function.

The subject of this column is who would take and be better for ginseng or red ginseng. I am going to explain jue ming zi (semen cassia) to understand better. Cassia is well known as a medicine better for brightening eyes. According to the old book, cassia is written sweet, bitter and cold. It is also moist in nature. It enters liver channel to clear heat, drain fire and brighten the eyes for eye problems due to wind-heat or liver fire blazing up. In order to use cassia for better eyes in case of no heat in liver, we must transform the property of cassia instead of using as it is. The method is to put cassia in the frying pan and make hot. This neutralizes the cold property by the heat. Most consumers are unaware of this fact and drink cassia tea and feel somewhat tired. These have no liver fire. If you believe and follow some idea without professional help, you may be good or can be worse depending on the individual.

Some book suggests Shaoyang constitution not to use ginseng. As Shaoyang in 4 constitutions has a body with a lot of heat, the use of ginseng is forbidden. As I mentioned before, red ginseng add heat into fresh or dried ginseng. It is common sense that adding heat on already warm nature will make warmer or hotter. There are some reports that red ginseng doesn't make heat, but I don't believe it personally. That's why some takes red ginseng for a long time complains palpitation, insomnia, indigestion, high blood pressure, and headache.

TV reported some people shows improvement and some don't. Let some who don't respond to try to take vegetables with red ginseng, then start to show improvement. I am not familiar with the word like Saponin and don't know at all how this substance work. However I dare to say that this kind of research institution doesn't know the basic of oriental medicine.

The basic acupuncturists know is yin and yang. In most cases it is desirable to balance yin and yang. Ginseng is an herb belonging to yang. Therefore ginseng is good for yin type person, but not for yang type person. Yin type person means cold body in general and yang type is whose body is warm. Think about it. Don't you feel it is desirable for cold body to take ginseng? Let us think about vegetables. Most vegetables belong to yin type. Yin type means cold nature. It is common sense that yang type person taking yin type vegetables are better choice. If yang type person take vegetables to force taking ginseng, it may help a little. Strictly speaking the study doesn't show which causes better between from ginseng or vegetables. However can you recommend ginseng in order to enhance yin type person with vegetables? If you don't know which type of body and take ginseng believing unconditionally making better, it may rather be a waste of money and harm your health.

These days the popularity of red ginseng is so high. So many patients choose red ginseng instead of visiting acupuncture clinics, the income of clinics decline accordingly. Some male patients who want to increase their energy switch to other drug like Viagra. Oriental collages produce lots of new students and the competition is so severe and many existing clinics are forced to close in Korea. The situation in U.S.A. is not much different. Once oriental medicines are most popular majors in collage, but now fall back to medium high.

Ginseng and red ginseng are a big help for cold or normal body type. The problem is ginseng may rather be harmful. There are a lot of medicinal herbs which can replace ginseng or red ginseng. I personally use dangshen instead of ginseng. I believe removing body heat is better than taking red ginseng.

ATOPIC DERMATITIS

This makes really sick for parents who have children suffering atopic dermatitis. The symptom improves for a while with treatments and relapse. This repeated cycle everyone crazy for children who suffer and parents who have no choice. The first thing is to know and treat what the cause is.

CAUSES BY WESTERN MEDICINE

1. Xeroderma

2. All stimulants
   Soap or detergent, disinfectant(cholorine in swimming pool), a stimulant in the work place, substance causing allergy through contact or airborne, dust mites, pollen, mold, hair dander, microorganisms, viruses and other

3. Mental factors (emotional stress)

4. Others

Climate (too hot or cold), hormones, exposure to cigarette smoke, irritation clothes, too frequent bathing, using electric blankets, and wearing too many layers clothes

COMMON SYMPTOMS

1. Family history of atopic allergies in the past

2. During infant, similar persistent eczema occurs on the head, face, body and limbs. At the same time occurs in the armpit and in the knee region folded.

3. After infant period, relatively well-site is on the face, neck, armpit, inner elbows, wrists and knees folded.

4. During childhood, adolescence and adulthood this changes to pityriasis making locally thickening and reddening.

5. Severe itching makes wound after skin scraping and causes secondary skin disease.

Above information are from the internet.

ORIENTAL PERSPECTIVE

Western medicines study the cause from various angles. Oriental medicines try to find the relationship with organs from the symptom. What I observed and found is that the skin becomes red and small rashes like heat rashes are shown. Then for whatever reason patients keep scratching. If you scratch, it becomes cool temporary. Everywhere are itchy, on feet, legs, hands, arms, torso, neck and head. Itching happens on whole body.

The fact skin color becomes red means evidence that the body has a heat. The ambient heat usually consumes the moisture around. When you enter the dry room, you may experience the difficulty for breathing. Sooner or later the skin starts to dry. Another example; if paddy field become dry, the bed cracks apart. It looks just like turtle top. This kind of phenomenon appears in the skin. While red skin turns into white color, flaking skin like dandruff start to fall.

Why do fetuses have more fever? This is related with the date of pregnancy. The date of pregnancy will affect a fetus. If a pregnant woman drinks lots of cold drinks and foods during the summer, the unborn child may have cold stomach affected by cold foods. If someone takes hot foods without knowing her constitution, hot foods affect the fetus. The fetus may born with hot constitution and increase the chances to expose to atopic skin.

TREATMENT

Some TV station reports the elimination of the atopic dermatitis on nature-friendly condition with natural diet in South Korea. In Germany some patient told me the experience that the patient was hospitalized and got treatments with strict diets provided only from the hospital for 3 weeks. The skin becomes very clean for the first six months and gradual recurrence returns after 6 months. There is a similar place in Japan, but far from the cured. This is the story what I heard from my patients.

The best treatment is to eliminate the body heat. Acupuncture theory tells that the skin belongs to lungs. There are cases that good improvements just by lowering skin temperature. Every acupuncturist knows about this.

However the problem is this alone does not solve the issue. Most treatments focus only on symptoms and try to relieve symptoms. The real issue is what the real root is and what makes lung hot or dry. This is fundamental, isn't it? It is difficult to say the complete recovery without recurrence. However my standard is to reach for at least one and half year or two years. If patients are careful with diets, it is possible for no recurrence.

I could cure the patient less than 16 years of age within one month. It is possible to treat more than 16 years old within one month, but some cases take two months for 3 times. As getting older the body may have accumulated increased drug use such as steroids. My guess is that's why it may take a little longer time. I suggest one month's herb medicine and acupuncture treatments of three times of a week for one month. Most cases take less than 6 times. If the treatment for the first month is not successful, I treat next month on me. If the treatment is not successful during two months, I may return the money I received. This guarantee applies only under the age of 16. This means I can treat this atopic eczema with a confidence. This is not the disease for you to carry a lifetime.

Let me tell you what foods must be careful with atopic dermatitis. In mild case some patients get benefit through dissipating the heat out of the body. But as the fundamental problem is due to the inner heat, the right method is to eliminate from the inside.

But the problem is in the milk.

1. Have you tried warming milk in the microwave? A skin forms on the top of the cup making reluctant to drink this film.

2. Let us boil the water and the milk in the same amount into the pot with fires of equal intensity. While the water pot vapors through the lid, this makes loud sound with the lid opening and closing. On the other hand the milk pot doesn't make sound as the lid is up and down on milk form of bubbles. A lot of milk drinking creates a kind of screen to prevent heat dissipation.

3. When drinking lots of milk, a form of film is made on the body skin. This form blocks the heat dissipate making to stay under the body skin.

I also recommend to refrain foods producing lot of heat; spicy food, lamb and goat.

Some patients get some helps from refraining milk, eggs and peanuts etc. Bible warns not to eat fish without scales; such as crabs, lobsters, shrimps, mackerel and saury. Roasted seaweeds may cause these atopic symptoms due to severe oxidation.

I had a chance to treat 2 years old baby and recommend avoiding the milk. The mother told me not to worry about that as she gave the breast feeding.

As the baby was young and I couldn't use herb medication, there was no improvement. I discovered the mother was a heat type of body and suggested to stop breast feeding as the baby eats other foods relatively well. The condition improved as the heat from the mother doesn't pass to the baby.

I am going to give you a great tip for you. Buy a stamp needle or seven star needles. Tap this needle into the subject skins. This will relieve the trapped heat.

Toothache

Having good teeth is one of the five blessings and a tooth is one of important bones. Before I became an acupuncturist, I went to the dentist against toothache. This is a natural conclusion as the dentist is a dental professional. I have thought for a long time how to prevent dental problems after couple teeth pulled out. My thought is changed a little bit now. When we follow the dentist advice, there is no option as dentists kill nerves or pull a tooth. I believe there are lots of people who got the proper dental treatment and experienced the shaky and painful bridge when the time passes. This is exactly what I experienced. That's why I gave a thought how to do by inexpensive way to treat toothache without removing a tooth. Do you think it is possible? Yes, this is quite true.

Let me tell you the conclusion. It is because of poor blood circulation around the gum. Pain around the gum is due to less supply oxygen and nutrients into painful area. When blood circulation is well, the pain will disappear and there is no need to pull the teeth. Of course there is some difference in certain cases. If the tooth is too loose, there may be no option except to pull out. However it may be more effective to treat it by yourself for a little pain or swollen one. This is possible by a single treatment. There is no need to kill nerves. If the nerve system is removed, this tooth must be removed at some point in the future. If the nerve is killed, the pain disappears. But lack of nutrition feeding into the tooth leads pulling out ultimately. The recurrence is the matter of time without improving the proper blood circulation. Even though the pain is gone after dental treatment, it is essential to prevent the future recurrence by better blood circulation. Meanwhile, it is necessary to allow the scaling once a year.

HOW TO TREAT NERVE WITHOUT KILLING

The laws of economics would get the maximum value with the smallest price. Using this law, I will show you how to treat toothache. This does not cost arm and leg at the dentist office. According to my toothache experience, the dentist takes X-rays to find the dental status where the pain is. It looks dark around the fang or tooth root on most cases. At this point the dentist advices us the treatment to kill its nerve. The cost is not cheap at all if you experience it already. This dark part is formed due to the poor blood circulation.

The simplest way is to find where the pain is by a finger pressing. After you find it, you prepare a sterilized needle and prick the painful area 3-5 times. Close the mouth and try the form to suck out and repeat a few times. The blood will come out through needle holes. Spit out blood and saliva in the mouth. The color of blood may be dark instead of red. If you repeat this procedure couple of times, the blood coming out will stop. I don't believe inflammation to worry, but if you are concerned, please rinse your mouth with salt water. You will find in the next morning toothache gone. If you still have the pain in the next day, do again. After you do this three times and does not work, you should go to the dentist. One of my patients who had an appointment for a root canal did the job on his own. He saved $2500 and thanked me very much.

WHAT HAPPENS TO MAKE A HOLE TO THE BONE?

I went to the dentist due to a loose tooth. The dentist examined and advised me to pull out a loose tooth and need a new dental implant. I answered him as I am an acupuncturist and I don't want an implant. What is got to an implant and an acupuncturist? I think this is a fair question, so I answered him that an implant will weaken the bone. He answered to me that the implant will make the bone strong. On hearing this, I changed to a new dentist.

I am not a dentist. But I cannot agree with that idea that an implant makes a strong bone according to acupuncture theory at all. Dental implant is the technique to make a hole into the bone and build up a screw and create a new tooth. I am talking about the old method as a new method developing every day. There are nerve issue and bone marrow inside the bone. For example when you boil the part of ox leg, the soup turns white color like milk. The surface that the leg cut shows lots of porous. Bone marrow is carried by these porous. Apparently the bone marrow should be flowed through porous. The hole for an implant will break nerves and block or impede the flow of bone marrow in the inner jaw bone. Based on this common sense, even though the jaw bone may be strong enough at the time of the treatment, the bone will start to weaken from the right moment of punching.

Many experiences with loose implant as the time pass by. I believe the above explanation is the reason. Acupuncture theory says kidney governs bones. Therefore kidney function will get worse also as the time pass by. I prefer a denture to implants. I recognize that all recommendations from dentists always are not good things after couple of teeth came out. I must admit many advantages of implants. However the price of implants is much more expensive than dentures. Money is one thing, but I still prefer dentures as I don't want to damage kidney. However whenever I eat foods, there is inconvenience for me to clean a denture. When you reach to the age needing implants, you may have a difficulty to digest hard and chewy foods. Please note that it is difficult to improve kidney function even by acupuncture treatments. I also recognize that dentist's opinion may be different with mine.

HOW TO STRENGTHEN THE GUMS AND BONES

I recommend acupuncture treatments for those that have already implants.

If better blood circulation is achieved, this helps gums stronger, but also the passage of creating bone marrow. This also helps to prevent bone inflammation. If the passage of the bone marrow is not free, nutrients do not feed properly the bone and the bones will be contracted eventually.

Do you know how the tooth pulled out left outside for a long time? It is the same reason for withering. You paid a lot of money to make implants. Now it is a time to maintain well. You need regular checkups, but also acupuncture treatments. We all need to become a little wiser.

Most people don't know organ problem affects teeth condition. Unless organs maintain well, it is unavoidable to have toothache. All bones belong to kidney, so teeth belong to kidney ultimately. Stomach and large intestine also affect a great deal to teeth.

Makeup and acupuncture

Everyone wants to look beautiful. Among them women pay more attention. Where represent the beauty of women most may be the face. While men use just the lotion, the vanity or dressing table of women is usually lined with various cosmetics. Many women have a faith that more expensive is better, so they invest tones of money in cosmetics and this is quite normal . . .

External factors creating dry skin

1. The first factor is lack of water; drinking water is important to maintain humidity.

2. Cold weather will cause. Cold wind in the winter makes skin rough. It is necessary to cover the face.

3. Hot heating makes dry skin; use a humidifier.

4. The sun is the root cause to make everything warm; refrain from the direct exposure to sunlight while going out.

The above cause is easy to understand and the solution is relatively straightforward. Aqueous cream is a good choice and face mask for moistening.

The cause from inner body

The major factor for dry skin is the heat from inner body in addition to rapid temperature changes. The nature of the heat consumes the moisture around and evaporates. Where the most heat is shown in common is the head. There are two important meridians. One is yang meridian and the other is yin meridian.

Yang meridians reaches to the head and yin meridians do to the chest. Yang meridians are pathways to carry the heat.

If there is something wrong with yang meridians, more heat is supposed to gather in the head. Therefore the oriental medicine claims the healthy condition is by the cold head and warm hands and feet. The heat in the head should come down to lower body. If not, this heat causes to dry facial skin.

If we strictly analyze the heat, this can be divided into two. One is excessive heat and the other is empty heat.

I mentioned already the heat has a tendency to consume the moisture around. When the heat resides on the face, the heat dries off the moisture and the face becomes dry. This turns eventually into the dry skin.

The problem does not stop only to dry skin. As soon as the face loses moisture, kidneys work harder for replenishment. This is because kidney is the organ that takes care of water. Kidneys do work hard and endure to some extent. However over time if there is no one to help, kidney will reduce the part of his job. For example kidney will send the reduced amount of water in the face. This leads to wrinkles. If anyone has a dry skin on the face through this progress, try to suspect weakening of kidney function.

Let me give an example with a tree. Tree roots are equivalent to kidney. In autumn leaves start to fall. Why? Trees protect themselves by minimizing the water to branches, as they know they become tired if they send the water even autumn and winter.

Important meridians to face are the large intestine and stomach. The constipation in particular is the main cause of the dry skin. The next one to consider is the heat of the stomach. There are many reasons of the stomach heat. One cause of the heat is from the start of diabetes.

TREATMENT

It treats just phenomenon or symptom to deal the dry face with cosmetics. But the real cause remains the same. It will look good temporarily with cosmetics, but it is better to find the real cause against the dry face. The reality is without knowing this fact and buy expensive cosmetics. This is a waste of money.

Consequences from eliminating the heat by acupuncture treatments are

1. The body becomes in balance.
2. The skin improves.
3. Savings in buying less cosmetics
4. Saving time to take care of dry skin
5. More time to invest on other important things
6. No worry about the dry skin
7. Prevent wrinkles in advance

You will become the real beauty in skin

If you experience the dry skin for a short period, it is possible or easy to take care of eliminating stomach heat, large intestine heat or constipation. However if these are long-lasting ones, it may require herbs. The principal of all treatments is the same. It is the best to fix it as soon as we find.

Please note that you have to think about the cosmetics by using nanotechnology which can reach deep into the skin. Comparison between inner and outer skin must be considered. The inner skin must be tender than the outer skin. This nanotechnology can change the color of the outer skin, So it may be chemically strong enough to adversely affect cells of body. While trying to facial care, it is possible to harm organs that are more important than the outer skin.

OILY SKIN

In contrast some suffer from oily skin. These may belong to Shaoyin based on 4 constitution theory. Shaoyin constitution is usually strong in kidney and weak in spleen. Kidneys are the organ that produces essence. As kidneys are strong, more essence is produced causing oily skin. Old books suggest not to sedate kidneys. Therefore in this case it is better to strengthen the spleen.

Finger arthritis, stiffness, wrist pain (Carpal tunnel syndrome), or tingling

Almost all things are done by computers these days. Many tap on computers more to work. There are many diseases on wrist and fingers. Some who go to church often try to write Bible by hands and suffer on hands. It is particularly noticeable to who engaged in occupation with a lot of strain on the wrist.

These symptoms on hands and wrist happen when you prepare kimchee or squeeze floor cloth a lot. These show tingling, numbness, swollen wrist, general pains, severe pain on catching something and unable to lift. Arm may be painful as well. Some does not grip the tight fist and may be not able to hold even a telephone handset.

Cause by western medicine

1. Symptoms accompanied by diabetes or thyroids
2. Depression of cervical 7 nerves connected neck and hands

Cause by oriental medicine

1. The beginning of all pains starts from the lack of Qi and blood. The pain means less oxygen and nutrition on specific local area. If you define the pain this way, don't you feel a little easy to solve the problem? As expressions like numbness or paralysis means due to poor blood circulation, this proper blood circulation alone is able to solve most cases.

2. Most finger arthritis followed by chronic progress rather than acute. Oriental medicine names wind-dampness and

rheumatisms known as western one. Knuckles become red as accompanied by heat. As the bone is governed by kidney, yin deficiency must be treated.

TREATMENT EXAMPLE 1

Everyone's pain may be different, but this person's pain is only on the third finger on the left hand. Her finger can't bend. When she tries to bend her fingers, all fingers are bent without the third finger. Those living in the United States understand very well what it means. This means "fuck you" for those who do not know. Imagine the scene holding the middle finger during a conversation to the other party. This is an insult to the other party causing lots of interfere in her social life. Those who know her understand her problem, but she had to describe her condition to the other party before they enter their communication. This is very uncomfortable to show her weakness. Because of this the topics of conversation sometimes flow to wrong area. So she figures it out to put her left hand behind her handbag. There is no guarantee even after a surgery. After I give 4 needles for a treatment, I asked her to bend her middle finger. The finger slowly starts to move with hesitance and touch the palm completely. She cried saying she didn't expect this. A complete recovery has been achieved after three next treatments.

There are cases stubborn on only fourth finger or fourth and fifth fingers together. There are surprisingly many people who suffer from this kind of problem. Good news is this is well treated by acupuncture treatments.

One acupuncture treatment could make two fingers bend by 60% for an American who was 71 years old and his hands were crooked more than 15-20 years. This man really was amazed by that. How is this possible with only 6 needles? He was amazed and repeated couple of times. If you know anyone who suffers with these symptoms, please let us know.

TREATMENT EXAMPLE 2

There are a number of ways to treat the pain in the wrist. I introduce the comparison between the surgery and acupuncture treatments. The cost of the surgery is $12000 and acupuncture is $1200. The result of both is satisfactory on either way. The surgery alone is not the answer. The cost of acupuncture is one tenth of a surgery. Personally I treat 2-4 times on most similar cases.

TREATMENT EXAMPLE 3

Knuckles of fingers are red and swollen. She works in sauna and has an economic hardship. She asked me there is any way to cure without acupuncture treatments. As she works in the hot place, she feels knuckle being affected more by heat. I advised her to soak on the cold water once in a while to remove the heat. She did this whenever necessary and was able to do this as the place is full of water. The red color disappeared and the pain and swollen hands also subsided. Treating the hot by the cold is the principal of oriental medicines.

More aggressive approach is poking the center of red area with a needle. Try to make bleeding from the outside toward the inside center by pushing and sliding. If you repeat this several times, the pain and swelling and red color will disappear. It may be easy if you think simple, but if you think difficult to fix it and worry only, the condition will become worse. Please do it now.

IS THERE ANY OTHER METHOD?

Soak hands into the basin containing hot water and a little wine with a little vinegar.

WHAT FOODS ARE GOOD FOR NUMBNESS?

Mustard, pepper, chili and etc. which are spicy are recommended.

NAIL RINGWORM (NAIL TOENAIL FUNGUS)

There are fingernails and toenails at the end of fingers and feet. Here is the meeting place of arteries and veins. Many people know nails as bone, but it is keratin. The reason for nails is to hold objects well. It may be difficult to hold or catch with flash alone. Most don't realize how serious fungus toenails are, as sucks cover toenail fungus and others can't notice at all. However this is a sure sign that a serious disease progresses.

SYMPTOMS

Nails changed to thick or thin and the color changes to yellow, black or white. This change shows some corner of nails or center only or entirety. Some types are friable form, show horizontal lines, or like mountain and valley or recessed pool and etc. Most happen only on one or two nails, but sometimes result in all 10 toes. One feature is that there is no pain. If there is a pain, everyone would receive treatments. But unfortunately as there is no pain, most is just to leave as it is without proper treatments. One young patient has all ten toes are black in color. He has never been swimming or sauna as he is afraid of showing his ugly toes. Some woman may hide nails with dark pedicures.

Fungal infection is called in English, but I don't think fungus related. The answer is on foot nails. We usually wear socks with shoes, heels or sneakers. This is a closed space. If this is a fungal infection, the fungus must spread to next toes. In most cases one infected toenail remains as it is and do not spread to the next toenail. That's why I oppose the word of mold. If this is related with fungus, even funguses know exactly which organs are weak. Fungus wants to stay and grow at the related organ.

One thing I can tell is this progress takes considerable amount of time. The color is light in the beginning, but over times the color changes into dark. In other words, the deeper the color is the more intense in diseases.

Treatment by western medicine

MD uses Lamisil, but the side effects are serious. MD sometimes recommends pulling out. Laser treatment turns nail color to white and sometimes fungus toenails are gone. But the problem is when the new nail grows over times; the recurrence follows in its original shape. This means the only visible symptom is temporary removed, but the real cause remains the same.

Traditional remedies

There are a few methods such as using vinegar, but the fact is nearly all cases recurrent.

Oriental concepts

The normal is pink. All other colors are abnormal. I mentioned before the relationship between organs and other body parts; liver: nails, heart: face, spleen: lips, lung: skin and kidney: head hair. Therefore I can assure you fingernails and toenails are associated with liver. But my textbook doesn't mention more than this. I had no way how to treat this toenail fungus.

I had a patient who got regular treatments. He told me happily six months later a black toenail was gone. He never expected how effective acupuncture treatments are. I had no idea what I actually did. Eventually I learned from the patient. Shortly afterwards I began to observe in details. I also did some experiments. For example if the patient who has toenail fungus comes with Bell's palsy, I treat Bell's palsy first. Even though Bell's palsy is finished,

I offer the patient free treatments for other symptoms. I provide acupuncture and herb on house. I did couple times. Some told that they felt the body lighter than before. Sugar levels in diabetic patients came back to normal. Some men who experienced incontinence and uncomfortable urination became normal. Some had a breathing difficulty even on not working, but after treatments there was no breathing difficulty even during hard jobs.

Through the course of this process I could find the relationship with other organs as well as liver and develop the principle of treatment. Now when I look at toenails, I am able to guess what kind of illness may develop in the future. But these names of sickness are often difficult to treat. Bell's palsy, stroke, diabetes, kidney failure, gallstones, urinary stones, cirrhosis, hepatitis, gastroptosis, stomach cancer, and lung related disease etc. are the sure thing, and there were many cases on hypertension attached with pace maker by heart disease. All are serious. This is a signal of serious disease coming. As fungus toenails do not accompany with pains, you may not pay attention. But you would better treat this as a dormant volcano. In many cases any bad symptoms do not appear in the test like MRI or CAT scan. You should not believe the result as it is, as these tests can't show everything. I explained why patients complain, but tests can't detect. The best is the prevention, as you try to treat later, it will be more difficult.

Please don't expect fungus toenails would be better immediately as soon as the treatment begins. When the body disease is treated and the body becomes well, fungus toenails will be gone automatically. Finger nails grow faster twice than toenails. As finger nails grow on three to six months, toenails grow on six months to one and half year. I have seen two years on severed cases.

We have to wait until new toenails come out from the root. You may expect thin nails in the beginning. On the next round the thicker nails come out. You can also expect the pink color of nails; this is normal color.

This is the solid evidence that this phenomenon is getting better.

TREATMENT EXAMPLE 1

This patient is a woman who looks too young for 70 years old and well educated. I noticed two black toenails while tapping needles. I asked a lot of questions if any other health issues or pains are. She insisted that she is healthy. I advised her to come for more treatments, but she didn't come. She felt sick and went to the hospital 3-4 months later. The liver cancer was spreader out to the pancreas. I asked her church member to let her come and get treatments, however she didn't answer the phone and cut off all contacts with outside world. Even though her son is a medical doctor out of the state, he was not able to help much either. All the words I heard were she got the anti-cancer treatment. I heard she passed away 3 months later. I emphasize again you may not notice any symptoms or pains, but when you feel it may be too late for treatments. Well, now you take off socks and check toenails. Husband does for wife and wife does for husband. Don't forget to massage feet each other.

TREATMENT EXAMPLE 2

This story happened to me. I had a slight pain on my right foot. I try to give a treatment, but I was curious how this pain proceeds. I left as it was as I am confident I can treat this kind one anytime. I observed almost daily how my pulse changes and the color of tongue. I didn't notice much difference. The pain had been remained. I treated six months later as the frequency of the pain came too often. Amazing things happen after that. The pain was on the right foot, but the left toenail began to change. Thin toenail began at the root and turned out to be recessed. It looked ugly. The front part is thick and new part of the root is thin. When the thin one grows to the front, the nail form was changed to be easily broken. After the treatment, the new thick nail comes out again. Even the pain was on the right side, but the symptom appears on the right side. I discovered one important fact. This is the actual experience which is not from books.

INFORMATION ACUPUNCTURISTS NEED

What causes the inside of the big toe is due to spleen and the outside of the big toe is due to liver. The second and third toenails are due to stomach. The fourth one is due to gallbladder. The fifth one is due to kidney and urinary bladder problem.

If the nail color is white, this is associated with lungs, if yellow color, with spleen and if black, with kidney. Other colors have not found with any particular association and problems.

All of these are caused by the liver based on TCM and the first treatment is essential to treat the liver.

HYPERTENSION

High blood pressure proceeds slowly for a long time more than 10years. When symptoms appear, this means some abnormality to some extent already to cardiovascular issue. It may occur rapidly within six months for young people.

The root cause of high blood pressure is due to improper diet and incorrect lifestyle on most cases. The root cause can be cured when we understand the root cause, doesn't it? The person who understands fast already knows how to treat. It is best to change bad eating habits and incorrect lifestyle. This may take a longer time, but this is the best. We should take more vegetables and fruits containing more fiber, various minerals, vitamins and phyto chemicals instead of meats. It is better to take vegetables on dark colors. Oriental medicine says that medicine and food have the same root (医食同源). Hippocrates said if foods can't cure, physician can't cure. This is the same meaning by either western or eastern medicine.

As hypertension develops slowly, it is important for early detection and checkup. Once hypertension is diagnosed, I recommend receiving a comprehensive medical examination once a year as well as checking up the blood pressure regularly. 140/90 and over was a high blood pressure in the past, but now 120/80 is considered as normal. However the current 140/90 doesn't go down easily as wished, so some suggests going back to the original.

The various complications follow by the hypertension. The cause of hypertension starts by narrowing of blood vessels. Narrowing means a smaller cross-sectional area of blood vessels. Higher blood pressure is required to send the same amount of blood. This pressure is hypertension. If you don't treat on time or neglect by any reasons, mild symptoms move to severe ones. If the reason of narrowing is by cholesterol, cholesterol will build up in the lining of the blood vessels. If the blood vessels are not provided by oxygen and nutrients, the blood vessels are going to die slowly. This is the process of hardening. Meanwhile as the heart works harder and becomes tired and this symptom persists, the complication of hypertension is to come. The heart muscle as well as all other organs must be supplied properly with nutrients and oxygen. If not, this is to be angina. In some cases the chest becomes stuffy and tingling or pricking.

The pain is very severe like splitting. In this case, most pain is on fixed place. In this case do not delay. It is the best to go to MD or acupuncture clinic at once. Acupuncturists may be able to remove or reduce the pain relatively easy without a surgery. So once in getting stuck you may remove the pain at first by just rubbing, but this is going to happen more frequent and you may start to think you are heading straight to die. While you receive acupuncture treatments, you can prevent further worsening by drinking tea we recommend. The tea we recommend costs less than 10 dollars for 3 months, so there is almost no burden. However a person who is older and whose pressure is more than 140 is recommended to take herbal tonic. We prepare herbs to consider the relationship between heart and other organs, so improve the function of the whole body. If this angina is not treated on time, myocardial infarction or coronary atherosclerosis is preceded by. When this happens, it takes more time to treat and costs more money. Prevention is the best of all diseases and the second is to treat earlier when the disease is light.

HYPERTENSION AND DIURETIC

When diuretic is commercially available at first, many believe the symptom of hypertension is over. As the blood amount causes the hypertension, many believe the hypertension would be resolved if the incremental emission can be made. Actually, and there were many effects from diuretic use. But over time, problems start to happen. Kidneys receive more water than blood required, so kidneys send a signal to the brain to pump harder more blood from the heart. This is totally unexpected. The scientists develop a prescription drug that suppressed the signal. Then the blood pressure becomes normal, but the function of kidney becomes worse. It is better to send more blood needed for kidneys than the suppression of the heart, isn't it? It is more desirable to consider all related organs than the symptom of the heart.

Many may be mistaken to believe just taking pills without knowing the fact. It is just like training a young elephant. While the elephant is young, a trainer ties the elephant with a strong rope to the very sturdy pole. No matter how the elephant acts, he realizes he can't move. Even he grows up and becomes so strong, as soon as he sees the rope, he gives up for moving. A lot of patients tie to the frame that they should take pills for a lifetime. This is not an exaggeration.

But many experience their becoming better in blood pressure with oriental herbal and acupuncture treatments. This is because not only treating symptoms, but also root causes with the relation of heart and kidneys based on the theory; heart is fire and kidney is water. According to conditions of patients, they consult with their physician to be able to reduce the prescribed medicine gradually.

HYPERTENSION AND STROKE

Everyone knows that the weather is colder in winter, but not many people know hypertension can become a big problem in winter. When the weather turns cold, every object has a nature to become shrinking. Our body is no exception. As the economy is not good, the winter is the season of shrinking with body as well as mind. The cross-sectional area of the blood vessel also decreases. The blood pressure will rise as the heart tries to send same amounts of blood into the reduced blood vessel size. When you have high blood pressure and constipation at the same time, there is a danger of cerebral hemorrhage when you try to push hard for constipation. So it is necessary to take care of constipation to reduce risk factors.

We heard once in a while that someone who goes to work early in the morning fell and paralyzed. This happens for the above reason. Anyone who usually has high blood pressure must be careful in the winter. MD advises taking anti-hypertensive for a lifetime. In other words the interpretation of this meaning is temporary effect. If you do not take medication, it will return to its original position. Since hypertension is recognized a few years after, a big pathogenesis will develop such as stroke and dementia etc. 95% of the stroke are caused by high blood pressure. Symptoms are stiff neck, dull feeling only on left or right side, or murmuring suddenly.

Although there are many causes of hypertension in oriental medicine, there are many ways to solve by oneself. Acupuncture treatments work very well and a lot better and effective with taking oriental herb tonic. There are some patients who take anti-hypertension to control severe symptoms and couldn't control or balance with heavy doses. When this happens, it is desirable to take western and oriental medicines. When you do this way the blood pressure starts to control. It the blood pressure goes down a lot (for example from 180 to 140), try to reduce the medicine amount by half. If it lowers again, try the amount to less than a quarter and stop taking eventually. When the blood pressure becomes normal, you are not required to take a lifetime. There are lots of patients who have done this way. The blood pressure of 225 before an acupuncture treatment fell to 180 sometimes and it took 30 minutes. Of course one treatment does not make to stay this way forever.

SELF-TREATMENT

1. It is important of salt selection. You should not take white salt which is relatively cheap. Make sure sea salt or bamboo salt. I think salt from Himalaya or Peru is good in theory. There is a salt mine of 80m deep with 800 going down stairs in Poland. This is also a tourist destination. These salts had created and made while not much pollution produced, so we can use safely. If you use this kind of salt, even taking

a little salty makes less problematic. I do not think the theory that salt causes hypertension is right.

2. It is important to take foods to prevent cholesterol. Everybody knows this fact; eat less meat and more vegetables containing more fiber. Take foods based on body constitution.

3. Increase the intake for onions, green onions and garlics.

4. Take more bitter taste foods.

5. Please refrain alcohol drinking, especially heavy drinking. Please note that caffeine raises blood pressure temporary.

6. Exercise

Everyone knows exercise is very necessary. However keeping is very difficult. The fact cholesterol covered in the lining of blood vessel is due to slow circulation. If you do not exercise, blood circulation slows down causing more buildup. However rapid or excessive exercise is not desirable rather needs to exercise longer and slower. The method may be a little different depending on morning or evening. The principle is related with the movement of the sun. The morning is the time that the energy rises due to the rising sun. The evening is the time that the energy downs. When you walk, put hands down in the morning and raise hands to the breast in the afternoon.

SECRET OF LONGEVITY IN OKINAWA

I love to watch health program in TV as I am an acupuncturist. As we get older and most people experience health problems, we just listen for a fun or try to learn something. I believe I may know more for health than the public. When I watch this program, I clearly understood more.

Okinawa in Japan is known for longevity. SBS broadcasted two series for that program. In the first broadcast they reported people in Okinawa take 18 different kinds of vegetables every day. Everyone knows eating vegetables is good for the health, so this coverage is not expected to be new. However there is a new content to the public which is taking a lot of pork. It is a little difficult for the general public to believe that pork belongs to the longevity food. The second broadcast shows bitter melon. This is unfamiliar to the public, but the appearance is like cucumbers. When you go to Chinese supermarket, you can find. It is characterized by very strong bitter taste. They also enjoy eating sea snake which is long.

While watching the broadcast I have a question. Where is Okinawa? I try to find through the internet, but failed. I forgot Japanese pronunciation as I haven't used for a long time. So I called my father who used to live in Japan. The answer is it is located at the end of islands of Japan and close to Taiwan.

The answer for longevity is already revealed. There is a Korean proverb called 신토불이 (身土不二). This means body and land are not separated, rather together. When we eat agricultural products where we live, we become healthy. Why?

The location of Okinawa and Taiwan is very close each other. I've never been to Taiwan or Okinawa, there must be warmer than where we live. It must be a sub-tropical climate. Therefore people born here are born with a hot energy. But most vegetables grown here belong to cold nature. The cold belongs to yin and the hot belongs to yang. Can't you see the balance between yin and yang? What about pork? Pigs are animals having cold nature. They have thick body fat to protect from the cold. This is the same theory. What about sea snakes? This is a kind of tricky to answer for me. The reason is the sea snake is not used as medicine herbs. In general snakes belong to cold-blooded animals. That's why snakes go into the warm ground in the winter for falling sleep. What about the snake nature that grows in the subtropical area? The original sea is considered as cold. Therefore fish that live in the sea is considered to be warm. However the temperature in tropical or subtropical ocean is thought to be relatively a little higher. For example the Arctic will be a little cooler. So the sea snake in this region is thought to have cool properties.

How do I interpret bitter melon? As the name applies, it has a very bitter taste. How would bitter taste act in our body? The action brings down the heat. A lot of sweats appear on hot weather or after exercise. Sweat is associated with heart with oriental medicine. Heart is the king organ in the oriental medicine. When the king becomes tired, all other organs become weak. The bitterness has a role to bring down the heat from the heart. Therefore if you eat the bitterness in advance, this bitterness makes the heart not to overact. People in Taiwan and India enjoy eating bitter melon very much. When you go to the supermarket, you may find someone who buys bitter melon and they are born in the hot weather.

After all no matter how wise man is, human beings are not better the natural order. In our view microorganisms and plants may seem to unwise, but as far as assimilating and living with nature, we can conclude they are wiser than us. Longevity may be simple; just eating plants where I was born. The truth is where it is closer, they say. This is a good example.

But we are looking for the good health in the wrong place. We just believe any longevity foods. Mediterranean diet is relatively easy to understand, but many believe Atkin diet which doesn't make sense.

According to the Mediterranean diet is almost vegetable-oriented. The meat is very small amount. This is relatively simple. Even though I deal with health issues, I am very confused with western approach.

Let me make a question. Would olive oil be good for us to Koreans? This is very famous health food. But it grows mainly in the Mediterranean. Italy and Korea are similar to the climate. It is similar with a spicy taste like garlic and pepper. But olive does not grow in South Korea. So would olive oil be good for Korean health? I don't think. Even though human knowledge is increased so much, we still can't ignore the principles of nature. I rather look for sesame oil which our ancestors have enjoyed. But I agree that cold press is better and more beneficial than hot press.

According to scientific findings, olive oil is rich in omega-6 fatty acid. Westerners love to eat vegetables with dressing. However as the smoke point is low, foods needed for boiled or stir-fry are not suitable due to more free radicals created.

Shingles and pain

Shingles is a disease that occurs mainly in adults. Shingles occurs mainly along the ribs. When a kid suffered with a chicken pox virus, this part of virus remains in the body and shows up when immune system is lower. Most complain burning, itching, and hot feeling and stabbing pain in some cases. It is very difficult to express this kind of pain and some wish just to drop dead. The reasons of pain are not known well, but according to the oriental medicine stabbing pain is accompanied by blood stasis or neurology, my guess is the pain may be related with them. Patients who complain pains rather choose to die consistently.

Treatment Example 1

This patient had shingles on the back of his neck. He was older than 62 years old. His neck was red and swollen and the thickness was about 0.5 cm. This lasted for 6 weeks. It made him hurt so much and he couldn't sleep. It was no use with medications of analgesic and viruses. He couldn't believe curing by acupuncture saying that even MD couldn't do how needles are possible. But his wife insisted so much and that's why he came. I told him as you don't trust the oriental medicines, so I am going to make you painful with needle inserting. He told me my pain is so severe and nothing to compare and asked me just make it happen. I noticed the red color changed to dark on the second visit, but no pain at all. He said this clinic's needle technique may be extra ordinary. When I explained all these happen due to lower immunity in the body, he ordered herb tonic for tonification. When he came to pick up the herb, all shingles are gone and many thanks to me.

TREATMENT EXAMPLE 2

One grandmother with shingles came from Uzpakistan. She took a prescription (steroid) from Russian doctor. This medication released the pain a little bit at a few times, but now it does not help her pain at all. She couldn't sleep a wink at all because of pains and came to the clinic very early in the morning with her son. When I observed the painful area, the skin color was green due to medicines. I saw a lot of similar one like urticaria distributed on her hip and thigh. Herpes zoster in common is shown on sides of the body or abdominal area and its color is red and very itching. But hers doesn't look like shingles. The patient was afraid of needles as this is the first acupuncture treatment. When I touched the tube containing a needle to her skin, her face showed lots of anxiety. I asked her "Are you ok?" She said "ok". At the moment she said ok, I gently struck on the top of the tube and removed the tube. She asked me why I don't give a shot. I told her it's over already. She has not been hurt at all. When she says ok, she is supposed to exhale. The principal of tonification in needle technique is to insert a needle while the patient exhales. Oriental medicine applies this kind of principal even on one needle. Although there is no principal of tonification or sedation in western medicine, oriental medicine has found of helping patients with long experience. When I checked her pulse a few minutes later, I noticed it normal beating. I asked her how she feels and she said all pains are gone. I asked her to recommend her relatives and friends about acupuncture and she said "Of course I will."

TREATMENT EXAMPLE 3—
HERPES ZOSTER WITH BONE CANCER

Shingles usually gets on one side of the left or right. It is mainly on the chest or the back and even in the face. The affected person typically complains stabbing pain like sticking pain by an awl. Skin redness and blistering is also common. She went to the dermatologist and diagnosed with shingles. She got about 30 blisters with the size of a split pea. The color is not red, rather dark red and the skin covered with a large gauze. Scraping of clothes is really painful. However this patient was during recovery with bone cancer. Her face was pale. As she doesn't have enough energy, she was very difficult to say a word. What was worse is where she got shingles is from the same area of the bone cancer. There may be a possibility of recurrence of bone cancer. My approach was very precautious. One of the characteristics of shingles is a lot of heat on the skin. So this heat leads to a red color. Her skin has changed to light color after two days later. She felt a little less painful. As blisters belong to damp heat according to oriental medicines, I gave the treatment to remove damp heat and blisters started to be dry. Blisters' scabs started to fall off one week later. Of course there was no pain either. I provide herbal medication to boost her energy as she had lack of energy after bone cancer treatment as I can treat shingles with acupuncture alone. Her face and chick turns to pink. She also feels more energy and starts the exercise. I also notice she does a makeup whenever she comes to the clinic. This is the evidence of becoming better with shingles as well as complication of bone cancer.

AM I A CANDIDATE OF THE NOVEL PRIZE?

One shingle patient got a complete recovery after three acupuncture treatments. He went to the pharmacist to return prescriptions; pain killers and antibiotics. The pharmacist refused to give money back and asked how it is possible for a full recovery after 3 treatments and said that acupuncturist must receive a Nobel Prize.

I will take it if they give.

CONCLUSION

Shingles occurs when the immune system is weak. Everyone knows about this. Then why gives only antibiotics and pain killers?

All I did was to strengthen the weak organs. I believe this is the right answer. As the immune system has weakened, the immune system must be taken care of. All symptoms have the cause. So we have to treat the cause. Am I right?

Why do women marry to whose age is older than themselves (oppa)?

Oppa here means a man who is older than a woman. The woman of marriageable age has a tendency to marry a man who is a little older than herself. Some say that the woman wants to receive a protection as man is stronger than woman. But everyone knows young man is stronger. Then why?

The interesting things happen in families who raise children. If you have a boy and a girl, the parent may notice girl is much more precocious than the boy. Let us assume a boy is just one year older than a girl. When the girl is four or five years old, she will begin to lead the boy. Even though the boy is older than his sister, the younger sister wins over her brother.

Ordinary people often observe this kind of story and think the girl may be smarter than her old brother. When the boy turns into the mid-twenties, he becomes more mature in appearance and thinking. This is the time most men complete military service obligations. So we usually talk that after man must go to the army, the man becomes mature according to the conventional wisdom.

TCM explanation

There is a bio rhythm cycle of the body. But men and women are different. The changing cycle of women is by every 7 years and of men is by every 8 years. Girls' hair becomes long and her tooth comes out at the age of seven. This kind of transformation takes place at the age of eight for boys. The menarche begins at the age of 14 which is equal to twice of seven.

When woman of age of 14 is equal to twice the age of 7, they experience of heaven water 천계 (天癸). This means the woman's first menstrual experience, menarche celestial. When an 8-year-old man becomes to the age of 16, equal to twice of 8, semen is created. Wisdom teeth breaks out at age 21 and the body rises to the peak. At the age of 24 the same phenomenon occurs on man. This means there is no longer in the height growth. She reached the peak on muscularity on the age of 28 years old and 32 years on a mam. The fertility began to fall from this point. In other words she is the highest fertility at the age of 28 meaning that it is better for the birth mother or the unborn child. When women become 35 years old, women start to lose hair and the face starts worn out. When women become 42 years old, the entire face is getting worn out and white hair is starting to change. This phenomenon is shown at the age of 48 years old for men and also changes the color of the beard. When women age is 49 years old, menopause arrives and the heaven water becomes the end to dry. As men age become 56 years old, muscle is weakened and moving around is uncomfortable. When men is 64 years old, semen is going to dry and teeth become loose..

THE ANSWER TO THE QUESTION

Compared with women beginning menstruation at the age of 14, men don't generate semen at the same age. A young man may look like a child to a woman. This relationship starts this way and continues to go. When women reach the age of 21 which can make a child by marriage, comparable age for men would be 24 years old. This is the reason women have a tendency to like and marry to men who is a little older than herself. In particular, we need to pay attention to the 24-year-old men age. This is the age men finish serving the army. Many people believe men become mature after serving the army, but the truth is this is due to biological cycles to complete a man. Even if many people give their opinions with unawareness of these biomarkers cycle, the real truth can't be found or difficult to answer.

There is an interesting phenomenon called romance gray meaning men who is 50 years or older might look for other women. This is my subjective opinion, but not related with TCM. Men may have a desire to thrive their children physiologically. But his wife's menstruation ends meaning she can't have children anymore even though he is able to do. This may be possible to interpret that even though the head understands that he should not, the body may look for the wrong way.

CURRENT IMPACT FROM OUTSIDE

Many parents surprise hearing girls less than 10years old start menarche. When we watch TV program with children, so many raunchy scenes are shown. While my kids were young, I used to tell them "Close your eyes a second." But the kids did not actually close their eyes. One mother complained TV programs. While watching TV with children TV showed lovemaking scenes. A son 10years old said "Mom, why does my penis surge?" She really didn't know what to answer him. She asked me how to answer. I recalled that as I was not majored in psychology, I don't know the answer.

WHY IS THIS HAPPENING?

There are too many visible raunchy things through TV and extreme miniskirts on streets. We experience that we don't know where we keep our eyes in the subway stairs. Woman's breast looks like see through and don't cover on purpose.

The bigger problem is from the food. Most meats on the market use the growth hormone. It would take 17weeks to grow chicken, but now takes only 7 weeks to make heavy chicken by using the growth hormone. Children who eat this chicken will be affected directly. I read some articles that female hormones are given to cows to make muscle soften as price of muscles like bovines are less expensive.

As most male pigs are castrated, unpleasant smell of fat from pigs are disappeared. Therefore there is far less chances to consume male hormone. Many men may become womanized due to the above reason. Many men may be eunuchs.

FUTURE PROSPECTS?

The question is woman's menopause will be occurred earlier or later as physiological function happens earlier than normal. Many young women under 40 years old worry about the menopause. In my opinion all engaged and worked in medical fields discuss this mater and prepare for futures. What is the reality?

Modern science proves acupuncture theory

It is difficult to believe the invisible things exist. Qi is the basic of all foundation. But it is difficult to measure Qi by modern science, so difficult to prove. Needless to say the spiritual world, too. However oriental medicine covers psychiatric problems, too.

Old book explains there are 5 different spirits in 5 zhangs. Heart retains the spirit. Lung retains the departing soul. Liver retains soul. Spleen retains the justice. Kidney retains the intention. The spirit is produced by the change of essence. Departing soul helps and rectifies the essence. Soul helps kidney Qi. Justice means memories and haunting. Intention means keeping the mind perfect and completely unchanging.

Old book explains the spirit is gathered by one male and female's essence. The departing soul hangs out and back along the spirit. Soul comes and goes with the essence. The justice means something to think in the mind. The existence of the justice means the intension. The intelligence is to handle things as intended.

Is this scientific? But interesting things have happened. Modern medicine has started to prove oriental medicine's theory from the unexpected ways. Here are some examples.

Case 1

There was a quite lady in quite nature in the country. She likes classical music and speaks quietly. She felt something wrong and went to the hospital. She was told she needs a heart transplant after the diagnosis. Fortunately she got the successful heart transplant. Her personality has changed after the surgery. She starts to love pro wrestling and rock music. Her parents watch her and notice this strange behavior. They ask her "Why does your personality change?" She answered back in return "What are you talking about?" As she was changed after the surgery, her parents asked the hospital whose heart was used. The hospital answered them this is the confidential information, so couldn't answer them. However this parent tries to find the donor's name and eventually got the address.

They went to that address and met the donor's family. The donor was a truck driver who signed "yes" on his driver's license to give anatomical body. His organs were sent to the necessary hospitals. His family testified he loves pro wrestling and rock music while he was alive.

This story shows the heart has a function of a pump to send the blood from veins to arteries after exchanging from carbon dioxide to oxygen, but also something else.

CASE 2

One pregnant lady came into the hospital. After careful diagnosis the hospital told her and asked her decision as doctors can't save mother and fetus. MD can save mother, but not the baby or can save the baby, but not mother. The family decides to save the baby.

In the meantime another lady came into the hospital. She needs a new heart. When MD has a surgery for the pregnant lady, her heart went to another lady. As soon as the lady with a heart transplant recovered from the surgery, she went to babies room asked the nurse" who is my baby?"

CASE 3

This man who is 60 years old has participated in all kinds of athletic contests and tries to receive diplomat of honor or trophy. His living room is full of displays of merits and trophies. However he was engaged in business so much and never interested in sports. He also cries on some female singer's song while he drives the car with his wife. All were happened since heart transplant surgery. His wife and friends couldn't understand him at all. His friends looked for whose heart was given to him and found from a stuntman. Who is the stuntman? They work on behalf of the scene that is dangerous for the safety of actors. How good are they in sports? Friends also found this stuntman loves that female singer.

There are more than 600 cases according to a scholar.

ARE ABSTRACT THE QI, MERIDIANS AND MENTAL CONCEPT?

In 1960 Kim Bong Han who worked as a director of North Korean meridian study in North Korea announced there are the third circulatory system next to blood circulation and lymph one. But this did not receive much attention in the scientific community. The reason for that was that the journals were not widely recognized. He didn't explain s how the experiment was found. Many scientists try to reproduce this reality, but failed.

Korean national cancer center have found the reality of the meridian recently. Using by staining technology and ultra-fine fluorescent particles the center observed the tube with a transparent color invisible with naked eyes. This tube may be a meridian. The center also observed this tube is the path of cancer metastasis and published in the international society. The center recovered the Primo pipe like thin thread.

There are 14 major meridians in the acupuncture theory. The one discovered this time came from Du mai. Du mai passes through the neck and the spine. If 13 other meridians and minor meridians are discovered, this will be a landmark discovery to overturn the meridian theory is not scientific.

I personally believed meridians. The reason is based on observing that the body becomes better for myself and other patients even though I can't see them. Now it is the time to argue whether there is meridians or not, rather how to use them. I believe this discovery will open another treatments as well as acupuncture effects. The best of all will be for acupuncture treatments.

It has been reported in Japan that there is subtle differences of the temperature measurement between acupuncture points and other parts of the body. Electrical resistance is less on acupuncture points than other parts.

The results are different: some are good and others failed with same colorectal cancer treatment according to TV Health Report. The founding was each person's genes are different. The different treatments by generic bases may be more effective, the report said. This is the same idea we call the constitution.

The basic concept of oriental medicine which was believed as fiction or unscientific becomes unfold by the rapid development of science. Now the concept of meridians was detected. I expect to detect 5 zangs store 7 different spirits in the near future.

I alone do this reasoning based on the above. As pigs have very similar organs with human beings, some scientists have a plan to transplant organs to human beings from no germ pigs raised by special methods. I presume it may be possible with liver or kidneys, but not with a heart. The reason is the heart is the king according to oriental theory. If this kind of the surgery is performed, this person may walk around with four legs. It is a personal opinion only.

WHICH IS BETTER EATING BREAKFAST OR NOT TO EAT?

There is a proverb called three in the morning four in the evening. One farmer raised monkeys. While there was a drought, the farmer talked to monkeys and was going to give them three acorns in the morning and four in evening due to this severe drought and asked them to understand. Monkeys upset very much. The farmer suggested the different way saying what about four acorns in the morning and three in the evening. Stupid monkeys became happy even though the total number is the same.

I think this proverb illustrates the importance of the breakfast. More seriously even monkeys know, but people do not know. This is my way of interpretation. There is one old saying: eat breakfast like a king, lunch like a minister and dinner like a beggar.

TCM recommends breakfast properly and formally in the morning, but dinner lightly like porridge. I heard a lot about this, but couldn't know why. Before I became an acupuncturist, I didn't know the oriental medicine just like you. So there was a time when I read or listen, if it makes me sense, it became a truth to me.

I watched TV program called The Great Birth Contest by accident. When an applicant sang a song, mentors on the bench evaluate about that song: song selection doesn't match with a singer or there was no color of singer singing. As I don't understand the music, I couldn't understand the meaning of the evaluation. There was a big difference between an export and a non-export. I think the same theory may apply for the health issues. So please listen to self-proclaimed export's opinion. However this may be a little difficult for those who do not know TCM.

I don't remember the exact time, but Mr. Ahn Hyeonpil wrote columns in the newspaper. I still remember his writhing that taking only one meal a day could eliminate accumulated toxin in the body, two meals a day remains the same and three meals a day means more toxin accumulated in the body. Early dinner and skipping breakfast means the stomach can take more rest and fewer burdens. He also recommended brown rice instead of white one. I had practiced for a long time as I believe it as the most feasible information.

TCM has a good theory that Mr. Ahn didn't explain on his column. When this theory is combined with his book, more practical theory will be born. This theory means Zhao Sporangia (自 午 流 注) concept.

Gallbladder	11pm-1am	Heart	11am-1pm
Liver	1-3am	Small intestine	1-3pm
Lung	3-5am	Urinary bladder	3-5pm
Large intestine	5-7am	Kidney	5-7pm
Stomach	7-9am	Pericardium	7-9pm
Spleen	9-11am	Triple burner	9-11pm

We call this as biorhythms in modern words. For example the time between 5:00 and 7:00 in the morning belongs to the large intestine. The time between 7:00 to 9:00 in the morning belongs to the stomach. In general most people get up at between 5:00 and 7:00 and go to the bathroom to take a bowel movement. Most people easily can understand this. The question is the time for the stomach. Some people say that they get the energy to work only when they eat the breakfast. However hours when foods stay at the stomach could be at least for three to four hours or five to six hours for the meat. These hours are only to prepare for digestion form, but not ready for absorption in the small intestine. This can't explain well how a person gets energy on what time with a breakfast. Some complain that they don't have a time to eat breakfast as they prepare to go to work. Some take only toasts and bacon due to the influence by the United States.

According to biorhythms, the time of small intestine is between one and three pm. After five hours in the stomach the foods are moved to the small intestine. The function of the small intestine is to absorb nutrients. When nutrients are absorbed energy, energy can be given to the whole body. After one o'clock, the sun energy starts go down. Even though the energy of the universe goes down, the upwarding function occurs in the inner body making yin and yang in balance. Nutrients absorbed in the afternoon will be used through the afternoon.

The time between 5:00 and 7:00 pm belongs to the kidney. Kidneys are organs representing water. TCM recommends eating the dinner like a beggar. Therefore the feast in the evening is not recommended. But how many people do eating the feast for the dinner? Most people overeat in the evening. Light meals are recommended like soup, porridge or smoothies. How many people do hear not to drink water in the evening as people experience the frequent urination at the night? This theory may seem totally different with the idea we are talking now. Many try not to drink a lot of water in the evening. But drinking proper amount is necessary to wash down the waste. There is a proverb saying "don't put off till tomorrow what you can do today." This is the principal that discharging all wastes must be taken out the same day or next morning.

Now, let us think another thing. What about the energy in the morning? Where does this come from? The time for liver is between 1:00 and 3:00 in the morning. Liver function becomes strong and voracious around seven o'clock in the morning. Liver has a nature of creeping up. When we have a good sleep, all fatigues are supposed to be gone. Therefore we have energy to work till one o'clock in the afternoon. Energy from small intestine would be used until the evening.

Now you understand the lunch would be used for energy from evening to the time to go to bed. This time is a relaxing time rather working hard like morning and afternoon. Therefore we are supposed to eat like a commoner as we don't need much energy.

Dinner will be responsible for energy during sleep. Most energy is used on breathing and blood circulation. Kidney is the representative organ of storing. Kidney requires lots of blood to store. You know growth hormone is produced during the night for young children. All are related with the function of kidney. However if we eat a lot of foods for the dinner in the late night, stomach takes out more blood for the digestion instead of providing to kidney. If the kidney is not able to store energy, the kidney is not able to nourish the liver. Then you may experience the fatigue and no energy when you get up and want to sleep more.

If we eat a lot of foods in the evening, our body might make more energy than we need. Where does this energy go? Accumulation of extra energy in the body is linked to obesity eventually

Therefore if we practice this biorhythm, we become healthy of course. Anyone who worries about the obesity will experience starting weight loss. Anyone who suffers from obesity doesn't have to stick to three meals a day. Look at the tiger. There is no fat tiger. If the tiger becomes hungry, it catches and eats. If there is no food to eat, it starves. In the past humans did the same thing. However we have too much and this is the real problem.

As there was no electricity in the past, I guess people go to bed early in the night. There is a lot more fun at night, so people go to bed late these days. Even though our life style has changed due to the science development, the function of body organs doesn't change accordingly. Now you understand the truth, why don't you go to bed early and save electric bills?

When I educate this information to my patients, they give me a wonderful feedback. There is a similar story in the India. Take a breakfast with all foods given to me, give an apple to the friend for the lunch, and give the dinner to the enemy, a grandmother told.

Here is one thing to consider. What about the person who works at the night and sleeps in the daytime? You can consider the time as the morning.

Living environment and preventive methods that cause cancer

1. External cause: damp heat
2. Internal cause: stress
3. Causes that don't belong to external and internal

According to some medical reports one out two would die due to cancer in 2050. The cause of cancer is too many to enumerate by western medicine. Some examples are toxic substances, chemicals, electromagnetic waves, infection by pathogens (the third cause). Everyone agree mental stress which is the internal cause.

When we look around, there are many people died with cancer who don't smoke cigarettes which are toxic substances, or try to avoid stress or live in the natural environment. From this point of view I begin to suspect other causes rather than the above causes. It is from germs in the air.

Herb leftovers

It wasn't easy to prepare tonic herbs in the past. Some remember hot stove made it worse on the hot weather to prepare on time and perspire a lot. The water was too much in the pot, so couldn't go to bed. Sometimes forgot the boiling pot and made it burn. All these problems are solved now as the clinic prepares them and makes them ready to drink in small plastic bags. This is very convenient for patients.

I put herb leftovers into the plastic bag and discard then on my back yards. Some told me herb leftovers are very good for farming and could be used as fertilizer. Some people ask me to collect them for their farming.

One interesting thing is the herb leftovers become changed in 2-3 days later. This change means fungus grows in the leftovers. The color of fungus is white, green or black depending on different herbs. All these happen due to germs in the air.

Another thing I have observed is the mold growth is different depending on scattered away or lump. The lump one makes mold grow fast. I believe this is the important point. The lump one means the air flow is less. Scattered one means the air flow is better. There is another thing I observed. Funguses grow from the area adjunct to vinyl bag and moves to the center in the vinyl bag.. In another words fungus grow better in the absence of oxygen.

The temperature of herb tonic boiling is 120 degree Celsius. It is so hot to touch as soon as the herb machine opens. After the herb becomes cool, the leftovers are discarded into the plastic bag. I have experienced many times warm inside of leftovers even though outside is cool. The most important thing is WARM.

Herb materials are dry before boiling, but after boiling herb materials are slightly wet: this means DAMP. I believe this warmth and dampness provide a good environment for fungus to grow. Herb leftovers may have lots of nutrients as well as a good environment. Microorganisms in the air seem to know very much where nutrients are.

BATH OR SHOWER ROOM

The bathroom must be warm as undressing is required. The door is closed for the privacy. The room must be warm as we may feel cold when we get out of warm shower. After the shower the room is filled with warmth and dampness. So the bathroom is the best place for mold to grow. You should see the green molds between tiles in the bathroom.

Western medicine explains when sweat comes out the body, amino acids company with the sweat making better environment for fungus to grow. What is the identity of sweat? It is the result of damp and heat. When the body becomes warm, the body releases fluids. TCM explains the sweat which is the body fluid from the heart is used to disperse absorbed heat in the body. The sweat out of the body would vaporize the heat around on the body skin. That's why we feel cooler after the sweating out. Even though there are some who sweats out every day, most people do not sweat every day.

But we use the bathroom every day.

TOILET WITH A VERY GOOD CONDITION FOR SPREADING GERMS

Toilet which has most germs is in the bathroom. Many of us experience to forget flushing the water after peeing. They also experience awful smell when flushing water next day. This certifies germs grow in the toilet bowl. What about the stools? I speculate there are lots of germs in pee and feces, especially from the patient. During flushing the water all germs may spread and fill the whole bathroom. Some of germs will go into the gargling cup.

One thing I want to emphasize here is to close the cover before flushing the water. If you flush the water with uncovering, there is a good possibility to spread germ into the air. Please make sure to practice this.

Most men urinate while standing. Men experience the urine falling out of the toilet bowl without exception. Many youngsters experience the morning erection when they wake up in the morning. It is very difficult to aim the urine in the center of toilet bowl while erecting. Even though some urine falls out of the toilet bowl, there are not many youngsters to clean or wipe the urine.

When men get older, the strength of urine becomes weaker. The urine falls out of the toilet bowl. After urination, men shake a penis to fall off the remaining urine. This action is no difference from a baby to men. This is one of the reasons the urine goes out of the toilet bowl.

The bathroom has an odor of urine in many cases. Why does it happen? As described above, the urine stays out of the toilet bowl. During the shower the dampness fills up within the bathroom. The bacteria in the urine combine with the dampness and grow causing the bad odor. Not only making the bad odor, but also ascending with warm air, so the nasty smell fills the bathroom.

There is no exception with women. Most female don't want to touch their ass to the toilet seat in the public bathroom. This causes the urine go out of the toilet bowl. In some case the toilet is wet due to this kind of action.

This is the reason why we have to close down the cover and flush the water after urine and feces. You are going to find soon that molds grow at the bottom of the seat and the cover. Therefore you need to clean more often.

GARGLE CUP

Let me tell you my story to make you understand better. There are a cup holder and soap holder on the top of the vanity. After I use the gargle cup with teeth brushing, I place it on the cup holder like everyone. This is a quite natural thing. I discover the color of the cup bottom has changed to yellowish. I thought this is due to chemicals deposit on the tap water. I try to clean the cup and look around anything to clean the cup. The only thing I found was a rag. I couldn't use the rag as my lips touch the cup. So I used my fingers into the bottom of the cup and rubbed on the bottom. It felt sticky. This is the evidence the fungus grow inside the cup. Even though I discover this fact, it is not easy to clean the cup every day. So I put the cup upside down. Since then there is no fungus growth on the bottom of the cup. Why?

After the cup has been upside down, the small amount of water was collected on the cup holder. The water becomes dry and the color is white.

This is the true color of disinfectant. Therefore if you see the yellowish or grey color from the bottom of your cup, this means fungus grow in there.

WHY THEN DO MOLDS GROW IN THE CUP?

Let us look at the cup. As soon as we finish the teeth brushing, we gargle and discard the water from the remaining water. However very little water on the wall moves or flows down at the bottom of the cup. If there are lots of water and the water flows and moves, there is less chance for molds to grow. However if the water is the small amount and doesn't move, this is the good condition for fungus to grow. Eventually damp is one condition. But when you make the cup upside down, the damp can't remain on the bottom. There is English proverb that rolling stone gathers no moss. Molds love stagnation and non-moveable place. Therefore molds are to require very little humidity or water. This is a very important fact. Of course the fungus belongs to bacteria.

The second is the house has the pleasant environment with almost unchanging in temperature. The bathroom is a warm place. We have to take off clothes to wash the body, so the radiator is absolutely necessary to make the bathroom warm. Warm or hot water is used for the shower or bath. While taking a shower, we close the door to prevent cold wind. After the shower, the dampness is filled inside the bathroom. This dampness companies with the warmth. This warmth is the problem. Bacteria or fungus grows better in a warm place. For example, when you put foods outside in the summer time, foods are spoiled in the short period. But the foods in the refrigerator last longer or spoil slowly. Many people experience that tiles exceptionally in the bathroom have molds. Now you understand why.

When you combine these two factors, damp heat makes molds grow better and fast.

HOSPITAL TOILET

Many people say when you visit or stay in the hospital, you may get sick from the hospital. I believe this has a significant base. Hospital patients may have more bacteria than others. Patients' germs in the hospital may be fatal and critical. These germs may move around easily through passages of heating or cooling. This is the reality on most cases. If people are not exposed to infection, this is not normal in reality.

If you go to some patients in the hospital, there are some bathrooms that have no lid in the toilet. Of course the lid of the toilet may be inconvenient for the patient. That's why the hospital gets rid of the toilet lid. It is understandable for the weak patient with no energy to open and close the lid is inconvenient. The best answer is as soon as the toilet is used, the toilet must be cleaned, but the reality is not easy to do this kind of disinfection.

When I tell patients about this, they watched this kind of situation from TV. When flushing the water, this water hits the toilet water and bounces back and comes out of the bowl. Bouncing back reaches more than nine feet, they said. Therefore my patients told me that they will make sure to close the lid in the future.

I read an article about the interesting test. Some mice were next the toilet bowl and others were at the laboratory for the experiment. Mice next to the toilet bowl die a lot earlier than others. What does this mean? I believe they die earlier due to bad germs.

Teeth brushing and fungi

Even healthy person may get 3000-5000 of cancer cells into the body daily according to western medicine. Where do these come from? Let us think about the path. After teeth brushing, we get some water the gargling cup into the mouth and gargle and spit and discard the water. If there are fungi inside the cup, there is a good possibility that small amount of fungus remain in the mouth and swallow. Our body has a good condition for fungi to grow.

The problem lies to people who have weak immune system and hate exercising and have a lot of stress. These people usually have less oxygen that is absolutely necessary. I mentioned already that fungi grow better where there is no oxygen. As the stress causes more adrenaline in production associated with the sympathetic nervous system, fungi make inflammation easily and will turn into cancer when advanced.

Environment and habits to be changed

1. Before you flush the toilet water, close the lid down to prevent germs spreading. You are going to find more fungi growth on the bottom of the lid and the seat. You have to clean more often to prevent germs growth. Try to choose a bigger toilet seat against touching the bowl while downing the lid.

2. Clean the gargle cup. Put the gargle cup upside down to prevent molds on the bottom of the cup. When you do this, you will find molds grow at the rim. Clean the rim and inside at least three times a week. Some use disposable cups. Some catch water by hands for gargling. The choice is yours.

3. After the shower, make sure to open the window, door or use a fan to remove dampness and make the room dry. If

the condition of the bathroom is hard to control dampness, please consider to use dehumidifier.

4. Make the shower curtain not to fold as folded portion remains wet and molds grow.

5. Dry toothbrush well. There are a few holes in the cup holder. Try to avoid the toothbrush touch the hole. Place it upright at the angle. Some says to put into the salt water.

6. Next area is the kitchen. The dish tower or sponge is always wet, so providing a good condition for fungi to grow. Put the sponge into the microwave and make it hot for two minutes to kill germs at least three times a week. If there is no microwave, boil with hot water.

7. The last one is the basement. Everyone knows the bad smell where the poor ventilation happens. Use a dehumidifier to remove the moisture. This is cold-dampness rather than damp-heat.

Cause of cancer-Stress

I mentioned already that stress is due to the change of the emotions. I can say confidently that most patients have lived under a lot of stress.

Confession of one female medical doctor

This medical doctor wants a long conversation with patients to determine the status of patients. She could see about 30 patients a day, but the hospital wants her to see at least 50 patients per day. If she doesn't see more than 50 patients, she feels the pressure that she may lose her job. She always worries she may misdiagnose due to seeing patients in the short period of time. Many people believe MD makes more money and some lawyers and patients are frantic to look for the chance to sue MD. If this happens, she may lose the license as well as whole property. It is difficult to handle this kind of fear. Let us think again about the stress one more time.

There are seven emotions in the oriental medicine. The above example is worry and fear. If she doesn't follow the hospital instruction, the emotion in this case is the worry she may be expelled. When she thinks about her young children in addition of losing the job, the fear becomes greater than the worry. Stress like this example relates very closely with emotions.

If this kind of stress persists, our body slowly starts to weaken. The so-called immune system will weaken sharply. Potential cancer cells inside will grow.

In this situation she got appendectomy. Since then her immune system sharply dropped. She strongly opposes the idea about the theory that the appendix is useless in the body. She believes the appendix is absolutely necessary for immune system because of her experience.

I don't know the sure reason from stress or appendectomy or the combined one, but I pay the attention on the fact of immunity fallen. Of course this is the universal fact that the immune system gets weaker. When the body is weak and cancer cells come into the body, the cancer may develop. When we are in good health, the cancer cells can't develop as white blood cells and NK cells can attack and kill.

It is important to reduce the external factors, but also to relieve stress quickly. Even though it is relatively easy to reduce the external factors, internal factors is not a simple problem.

As there are various ways to reduce the stress, I really want to encourage laughter. Be forced to smile. There is a legendary story that one person became sick. He rented comedy programs for one month and laughed for one month and all his sickness was gone. I heard there is a program to be a laughter therapist in Korea. So try to learn any way suitable for you and laugh more.

Laughter is related with the heart by oriental medicine.. And the heart is the king. When the king is strong, all servants become stronger. When you laugh more, a lot of oxygen will be supplied involuntarily to fight back against the cancer.

THE THIRD FACTOR OF CANCER

Lots of chemicals and pollution etc. are other factors. It is not easy to avoid these materials. If possible we just try to avoid and not to use risk factors. That is all we can do. For example we live in this world that we can't rule out all the chemicals even though we know the chemicals have some carcinogen.

EARLY DETECTION OF CANCER

The survival rate of 5-year is more than 50% if the cancer is detected earlier. Compared with the past consideration when we just die if we get the cancer, the condition has improved so much. But I don't think the survival rate has been improved because of improving the method of treatments.

In old days X-ray was used to determine the cancer. It was difficult to identify less than 3cm. We didn't know the start of cancer for even larger than 3cm. Therefore the date of the treatments was based on the date of discovery. It was difficult to pass more than two years at the past.

Even the size of 5mm can be discovered with the development of medical diagnostic technology. We know progression speed is different depending on the types of cancer. Assuming the cancer becoming the double size for one year, anyone can tell the big different size between 5mm and 30mm.

Let us calculate the circle area with consideration as a circle for 5mm and 30mm. Volume may be more precise than circle, but all cancer forms are not like a ball, so let us figure the growth rate. As the π is the common molecular, I calculate the size of 5mm and 30mm and their areas by deleting π. 5mm becomes to 6.25 and 30mm becomes to 225.

Number of years to be changed from 6.25 to 225

Year	1	2	3	4	5	6	7
size	6.25	12.5	25	50	100	200	400

We assume the size from 5mm to 30mm takes longer than 6 years. The five year of survival rate doesn't mean much at all. The survival rate of 50% looks giving us a hope numerically, but doing nothing without treatments takes for more than 6 years. This means some patients may die earlier after treatments by 50%. This is the reason why I think not because of improvements in treatments, but early detection.

There is no significant difference between that patients don't know the cancer and that early detection makes possible for a patient to live for five years. Even though there are several variables, if the early detection and suggested treatments couldn't save more than five years, patients may feel very unfair. I don't believe their quality of life has been nice.

I recommend patients to receive oriental treatments while taking western treatments. Early detection is desirable to use the wisdom of western medicine and the quality of life by oriental medicine.

Conversation with cancer cells

Some has discomforting feeling and goes to the hospital. The diagnostic result is the cancer. How do you react if you are like this case? This kind of situation has happened to a lot of people and is going to happen in the future. There is lots of good information how to cope with cancer in the internet. So please refer with them.

This is the typical example.

What is our attitude when we hear and find that the all examinations conclude that we have cancer?

- Some think this diagnoses may be wrong and try to go to different doctors.

- Why does this happen to me?

- Most become angry and start to accept about this situation, but only up to certain limitation like I have to live until children finish their education or marry.

- Some become depressed and lose their speech.

- We gradually accept to face it. We wonder, is there any hope for me? What is the success rate of surviving after the surgery?

All surgeries require cutting off the damaged part and lot more as no one knows how wide the cancer has spread. Once a part has been cut off, the subjected organ never grows back to the original size except the liver. The liver will grow back. What about other organs? Is there any other way to save the original organs?

I recommend considering all possible sources to win over this unfortunate condition.

CANCER CELLS ARE STUPID

Why do I say this? Cancer cells love to grow and spread as much as they can. When cancer cells grow too much and the patient can't live any more, cancer cells will also die. They are very greedy. They live for only themselves. They don't know they will die if their shelter is wiped out. That's why I call them stupid. Before developing this idea further, let us consider these stories.

THE REASON FOR POSSIBLE CONVERSATION

1. Please follow my instruction while you close your eyes. You go to the kitchen to look for something to drink. When you open the door, you see only lemon. You take out the lemon and cut it in half with a knife. You smell the lemon scent on your hands, oh, the smell is good. You make the halves into half again. Make a quarter pieces into half again. Pick a piece of 1/8 up and take this into the mouth and open the mouth and squeeze it on your mouth. Lemon water is high in the mouth. Now you open your eyes. You notice saliva due to the sour taste. This is the just imagination, but the actual saliva is accumulated.

2. We know mushrooms usually grow in a humid and shadowed area. They prefer a humid condition. Farmers sometimes play a musical raining sound where they grow mushrooms. Even though it is not a real rain, mushrooms grow better as they love rain.

3. Japanese scholar found that even water understands love or hate. When a human being says "I love you" to water, water forms a beautiful shape of ice. When we say "We hate you" instead, water forms ugly shapes of ice.

4. There are some people who can communicate with animals, even though human being and all animals use different kind of languages. This person talks to the animal and the animal talks back such as "when I was abandoned by previous owner, I should have died at that time, but I still am alive." When their new owner conveys that they really like the animal, through the interpreter, the animals' behavior improved because of this kind of communication.

All these stories mean that every organic being in the world can understand intended communication by potentiality and unconsciously. This means that even cancer cells will understand if we try to convey the true situation. It may sound silly to you, but I believe it may work. The approach may be like this. I am not asking cancer cells "You drop dead", or "I hate you" or "You devil, get out of me".

Rather say, "let us live together and don't grow anymore. If you grow too much, you will also die."

When I mention about this, one missionary replied this way. When we practice this kind of dialogue "how greedy and stupid", this may apply exactly to us how greedy I am and how stupid I am. When we realize how greedy and stupid, we can turn around our life style and thought, then we may recover from the cancer.

I want to hear your "best dialogue with cancer cells" from you who read this. Maybe a good psychologist will create a good dialogue. I am going to list here and your name or organization. Let us create a new method of cancer treatments and contribute something new to this society.

Attitude to cure cancer

Concentrating on something we like most.

Here is a true story. A father was diagnosed with cancer and it was too late for a surgery. The MD told his family that he may live only for three months. His daughter debuted in a TV drama around this time. He was very proud of her and wished her a big success. Her father loved her TV drama and waited for her weekend program. After watching the program, he monitored everything related with his daughter's role, and read all the critiques and opinions from other viewers. He also told all the other patients in the hospital that she is his daughter and asked the other patients to watch the program. A miracle happened after one and half months. His cancer size shrank to half and it was possible to do the surgery. The surgery was successful and he has lived more than five years now.

Who doesn't like his daughter becomes better? This man falls in love on his daughter. We should engage in something to love. We can call or visit our parents of family with sincere love and spend times with them. Or you can choose the mountain where there is clean air and water. We also can find the postponed plan and do this plan with a delighted heart. Another one is to devote to a religion. There are plenty of these kinds we may be able to do.

Breast cancer and Dry Ice

We also figure out how to treat this cancer: such as western medicine (surgery, chemotherapy, radiation therapy) as well as oriental medicine. This is my opinion only. I am all for the surgery, but chemo and radiation therapy must be considered seriously. There are some ways that are not approved in the United States, but in Germany. I introduce this as this method is not known well to the public.

I have one patient who has suffered with the breast cancer. Her primary care physician recommended her to go to Germany to treat her breast cancer. He attended a seminar in Las Vegas. The instructor from Germany introduced the new method convincing MD to recommend to his patients. When I heard the treatment from the patient, the principle of treatment is the same with oriental medicine. One method of oriental medicine is to make cold if hot and make hot if cold. As this patient had high fever, German MD injected dry ice into the chest. Dry ice is very cold as you know. This is a good chemistry between heat and dry ice. This story convinced me that Germany is one of the best countries with alternative medicine. Even though they may not understand oriental theory, they apply this principal with a different way. Since this treatment she had lived without any inconvenience for a couple of years.

There is another way to treat. If the cancer is cold, the treatment is used with very hot heat. Some cancer cells cannot survive under the condition of very hot heat. This method is to put the patient into the dome set with appropriate temperature depending on patient's condition. This is different way compared with radiation and chemo therapy.

I suggest you to consult with acupuncturist which method should be used. The reason is that acupuncturist can do better to distinguish hot and cold. The different outcome may be resulted depending on the selection.

GASTRIC CANCER GONE

One patient came to my clinic. He was diagnosed by gastric cancer after endoscopy and biopsy. He had two weeks of time before CAT SCAN and wanted to get acupuncture treatments during two weeks of waiting period. He also complained swelling on the face and legs and the fatigue. After acupuncture and herbal treatments for two weeks, his fatigue and swelling were gone. Herbs were used with reducing the stomach heat and tonifying energy.

He took CAT SCAN three weeks later. The scan didn't find any stomach cancer at all. MD who ordered CAT SCAN became absurd on the fact that no cancer was found. He checked the file and confirmed the cancer. He performed another endoscope and also found nothing three weeks later. He couldn't understand what happened during last three weeks.

Conclusion

When you hear that you get the cancer, do not panic. The most important thing is to have peace of mind and get treatments. In the meantime you continue conversation with the cancer. Most side effects from chemotherapy are nausea, loss of appetite, dry skin and hair loss etc. These side effects are well controlled by oriental medicine.

STEVE JOBS AND PANCREATIC CANCER

I usually joke that Steve Jobs successes due to his name. He created so many jobs like his name. Bill Gate is in the same boat. All bills come to his gate. No wonder he made so much money. Arm Strong is not an exception. His arm is strong, so he could lift and hold a strong trumpet and play music well.

When I read the newspaper that Jobs had stick to natural therapies instead of a surgery, so he died, I did feel something wrong about the fact. He was a veganism to overcome the cancer. If I treated him, I may be able to tell you all facts instead of my imagination.

I have not read his biography, rather on articles or memories from newspaper or internet. He used to eat mainly sushi at the restaurant. Everyone agrees that he works passionately until he dies. Even though he appears at the presentation with a lean body and many people were saddened, we have to point out he works without giving the company hindrance. If he had a surgery and lived more than five years, the surgery was successful according to the standard of the survival rate of five years.

His cancer was discovered in 2003. And he died in 2011. He had lived for eight years after the diagnosis of cancer. He may die earlier than 2011 if he had a surgery. This is only theoretical, but may be not totally wrong. He may be not able to work passionate with suffering by chemotherapy or radiation therapy. While I read newspapers about his death, articles were too biased against the naturalistic treatments in my opinion.

Occupy the Wall Street

Some protest and complain the inequality that one percent of people have 99% of wealth. When I watch this protest, this makes me think of the human body. This is the structure of the cancer we are afraid of. When the cancer is grown largely, the weight of the cancer is one percent of the entire body. I don't mean that one percent of people is the cancer, but only with a number. One percent of the rich people are not absolutely cancerous presence. By the way, 99% of the body will be affected by 1% of weight in cancer. Western medicine might focus on the 1%.

Chemotherapy, Radiation, and Surgery

When the surgery is performed, the cut is the visible part and much more. The reason is the cancer is like weed roots. It is relatively easy to cut the large roots, but no one knows how much the fibrous roots are spread. So in order to kill any remained cancer cells anticancer drugs and radiation therapy are used. I personally think chemotherapy and radiation therapy have some problems. The concept of western medicine must see the subjective with a microscope and this is to be considered as a scientific method. However invisible ones are treated by the strong conviction only by the above methods. That's why these treatments kill normal cells as well as cancer cells. This causes the side effects.

These side effects are nausea, vomiting, loss of appetite, hair loss and skin color change. Patients cannot eat well and become skinny. Some cases not only hair loss but also eyebrows. These are natural body reactions due to non-fit condition. This is the signal our body does not like these methods. My personal opinion is there is lots of room for improvement with these treatments. Most patients just accept these side effects without much complaint. If any patients vomit with my herb treatments, all will say this is something wrong and complain about the herb. I do understand this kind of reality as patients are not professionals without much knowledge.

Prescription drugs are prescribed as this anticancer is the poison and too strong and patients have a difficult to eat and vomit. Radiation therapy is very identical. We all understand the principle is to kill cancer cells, but also healthy cells. Even though there are state-of-the art machines to minimize the killing of normal cells, there are not many ones. All are ways to kill 1% of cancer.

As far as the surgery is concerned, I am entirely in favor. The surgery is the specialty from western medicine.

Oriental medicines focus on 99% rather than 1% of the cancer. Some cases report the cancer was removed or disappeared by the oriental medicines, but there is limitation to get rid of the cancer on most cases. It is possible not to grow further against the cancer. If you think the quality of life, the oriental medicine may be more beneficial.

It is relatively easy to treat vomiting by acupuncture treatments. Loss of appetite is well treated with Korean 4 needles. When the appetite comes back, patients must be able to digest. Then patients have energy back and strength to fight back and overcome against the cancer. I also experience taking herb medicine is a tremendous help for patients. I suggest getting oriental medicine to minimize the pain while taking western medicine. This should be significantly enhancing the quality of life of the individual patient. What good is it to reduce the quality of life for the purpose of extension of life?

If the cost is more than a few ten thousand dollars to prolong the life a few months, most families can't afford these tremendous costs of the treatment if not paid by the insurance company. On the worst case it could be tremendous burdens for the remaining family.

THE PROGRESS OF THE CANCER

In TCM there is a theory that yin changes into yang and yang changes into yin. For example the day changes into the night and the night changes into the day.

Let us think about the liver cancer. We understand the progress of the liver disease as follows: hepatitis, cirrhosis and liver cancer. The liver cancer doesn't develop in just one day. It took many years to develop.

This is my opinion. Cancer cells have development from hepatitis. The only thing is cancer cells are too small to see at this moment. Hepatitis is the condition that the liver temperature is warmer than normal. The heat consumes the moisture and makes it dry. When it becomes dry, it turns to hardening. (Please note some cases making heat to soft) This period is cirrhosis. When there is no longer of dryness, it becomes to get cold meaning liver cancer at this time.

On the other hand, the breast cancer seems to proceed in reverse. This begins with the cold and changes into hot in the later stage. Those who suffer with breast cancer have a relatively weak spleen and stomach.

As the progress is different, the treatment method must be different. What is your opinion?

In order to prevent liver cancer, what is going to happen during hepatitis if you take mushrooms? I mentioned the mushrooms have warm nature. The progress of liver cancer may develop further. For the breast cancer mushrooms are good for prevention, but not good in the cancer stage.

Without knowing the fundamental reason, we have to be careful to take anything; so called cure-all medicines or foods.

AFTER READING THE BOOK WRITTEN BY MR. KIM NAMSOO

I bought and read his book with an expectation for learning something that I don't know as he is so famous and has a long clinical experience. The treatment of burns is explained at the end of the book. I give my respect for the method for burns. I have never seen any patients of burns as most burning patients go to the western doctor. This information is not mentioned in the most books, so it looks very fresh to me. The method is to apply many acupuncture needles on the burned area. As I learn the new technique which can treat burns within from one week to one month, this information is worth enough to cover the book cost. If any patient visits with burns, I am going to use your way.

All other contents were not a big deal. It was just general contents all students in oriental medicine learn in school. All acupuncturists are able to treat shoulder pains, lower back pains or sudden indigestion. Your book informs many people that acupuncture and moxibustion can treat even impossible symptoms that western medicine cannot do. Of course oriental medicine can't treat all diseases, but your book opens up the good possibility to help in many diseases.

SIDE EFFECTS OF MOXIBUSTION

However your book doesn't mention about the side effects of moxibustion. As you know, points of acupuncture and moxibustion are the same. When we do moxibustion many times on the same spots, these spots cause small burns on the skin. Meridians which Qi and blood flow are similar to a pipe. As an impact on the aluminum can makes a dent, the scar on the skin would block meridians. When this spot must be used for acupuncture needles, we can't use the bull's eye of accurate points as needles can't penetrate into the scar. The only way we can do is to set needles aside the exact point resulting acupuncture effectiveness much less. Right needling is similar to shooting arrows. When we needle on the bull's eye, results are like ten points. When the arrow is beyond the target, no points are added. When we do many moxibustion on the same points, the small scar is changed to just like after the surgery. The order of treatments is the acupuncture is the first, moxibustion is the second and the herb treatment is the third, as we understand. However you emphasize the moxibustion, so my opinion is different with yours. Therefore some patients may complain that acupuncturists don't have the knowledge as the result is not good as expected. It is difficult for us to change the misconception of the fixed opinion.

Moxibustion is one of methods belonging to yang in yin and yang. This method is good for the cold body, but it should not be used uniformly to the people who have a lot of heat. Some patients who try moxibustion come to my clinic. They try the moxibustion, but the result was poor. One common thing is these people have warmer body than the normal.

The best way to use moxibustion is to burn mugwort. Put the very small particles of mugwort on the skin. Light the top on the particle of mugwort.

The particle burns from the top to the bottom. The burned changes into ashes, but ashes stay as it was. While the particle burns, the particles make blue smoke on the top and yellow smoke on the bottom. When the burning particle touches the skin, this yellow smoke gets beneath the skin. There is a method not to burn the skin by extinguishing the inflamed particle. There are several methods but not described here. As I understand there is no other plant leaves making yellow smoke. Therefore moxibustion is one of the ways to treat by the heat. This means this method is effective for the cold nature, but not for the hot nature in my opinion. I don't agree that there are no side effects to anyone.

GROUP FOR LOVE OF MOXIBUSTION

This is the organization Mr. Kim Namsoo has made. This organization claims that acupuncturists don't know well how to do the moxibustion. The true answer is we don't use moxibustion, not because we don't know. When burns mugwort, there is a bad odor. This is really like smells burning marijuana. Most clinics are leased. It is difficult to install the fan to exhaust the bad smell on most clinics. While burning mugwort, there is a lot of complaining from the upstairs, next rooms or next beds. Most acupuncture clinics have a police visit for the report the clinic uses marijuana. The patients don't realize how bad the smell is, but the next person may suffer with this bad odor. It is impossible sometimes for eye opening due to stinging air without using a fan. Even if the room has a fan in facility, the smell remains in the room when entering the room. This smoke also changes the color of the room paint. During the winter time, when we open the door, the patient herself feels cold. What about the next patients who don't get moxibustion? We just don't practice moxibustion due to these reasons. That's why it is not desirable for this organization to claim that they do better than us.

Before I read his book, I thought Mr. Kim Namsoo is a great man. When I read articles in the newspaper for free treatments for many people, I thought that acupuncturists in Korea are a little bit spoiled.

I fix the small plumbing job at home personally. I can save a lot of money if I can fix without calling licensed plumber. I can call the licensed plumber if I can't fix by myself, so who is going to bother about this idea?

Despite the fact moxibustion is relatively safe; it is quite natural to get bad mouth against acupuncturists who want to block Mr. Kim Namsoo for practicing moxibustion. So I thought licensed acupuncturists try to block free moxibustion services in order to keep their portion of the pie. I am a licensed in the United States. I don't say this as I don't have a license in Korea or not practicing in Korea and there is nothing got to with me.

As I have left Korea a long time ago, I was not interested in Mr. Kim Namsoo. I knew that the organization of Love of Moxibustion was found by him after reading his book. And this organization issues the individual license. I think this is not right. Issuing certification must be done by the recognized and state agency, not by the individual. I thought this certification is given free. But contrary to my belief, this organization charges $2500 per tuition. The articles that tuition alone was twenty million dollars made me awkward. He may provide free services or try to introduce the method requiring less money to the public. But the real purpose is to be a good business man, I wonder.

The most what he said is true. That is why many people cheer about him. They believe that acupuncturists are interested in their pie only. As you mentioned you are not interested in making money, the solution may be surprisingly simple. Moxibustion is really working effectively. Go the local acupuncture clinic and ask to mark points on the skin and start the moxibustion. This is the best way to build each individual health with costing less money. I don't think there are any acupuncturists objecting this idea. It may take one hour and cost $100 only.

One of your students in the organization posted an interesting article asking the acupuncturist to compete as acupuncturists have no skills. I want to ask you to refrain such reckless post. If you believe your student, I really want to respond and participate who does the treatment quickly and better. What about frozen shoulder pain, stomach pain, hypertension, atopic skin or acnes? I don't mind any symptom you want.

The motivation I wrote this was after the report concerning former President Roe Taewoo. The argument or fight between you and acupuncturists makes shameful appearance to the public. My guess is one needle was left on the side. Someone forgot to take it out. The patient tried to lie down to the other side. During lying down the other side, the needle remained went into the body. The needles used in the United States are designed that the needle can't go into the body. It may be useless to point fingers as this kind of mistake can be happened to anyone. One of ways to stop this useless argument is to ask patients to go to local acupuncture clinic and learn from them.

Sciences destroy the natural

The developments of science are able to make men to go to moon. When I was in school 50 years ago, I read an article that if electric lights are on in the chicken farm, more eggs are produced as chicken believe it is the daytime. What a brilliant idea was my thought at that time, but now I think differently. As chicken suffer with stress, they may produce very high amount of stress hormone. This stress hormone will be delivered into human body after all.

Bible commends not to eat the blood of animals as life is in blood. Scientists explain when the time comes on the slaughter of animals, they know they are going to die and produce lots of stress hormone at that time. This hormone will affect our body. Some claim Bible is not scientific due to the Copernican theory, but as far as human body is applied, this is very scientific.

Here is another example. The streetlights are very convenient at night. However plants under streetlights happen to suffer as the light is against nature. The laboratory tests show that the growth rate is slower under streetlights compared to normal conditioned plants. The production also is 10-15% less. If we eat these crops, plant stress may be accumulated in our body and affect us.

In fact, we are in defenseless state these days as we don't know how they are produced. How are you sure about your immune system without knowing all plants and animals stress? We must respond against this stress by acupuncture and herbal treatment as the stress may be the origin of all diseases.

Mosquito bite

When mosquito bites on our skin, we apply saliva or ammonia to reduce the itching by neutralizing the venom of the mosquito.

Let us think about the reason why mosquito bite make the skin itching. In old days, we call mosquito venom the evil qi. And there is the right qi in the body. As soon as the evil qi comes into our body, the evil qi tries to expend the territory in all directions. However the right qi are around the evil qi in order to prevent for the evil qi to penetrate into the body. The heat is produced as the result of the fight between the evil qi and right qi. The heat has a tendency of evaporating and consuming the moisture. For example when the water is evaporated in the rice paddy, the rice paddy starts to crack. The same action would occur in the skin.

If we try to explain this by modern science, white blood cells try to defend against venom. White blood cells surround venom. Venom tries to expend and white blood cells build the defensive disposition. I believe white blood cells have a spirit of an elite youth corps of Sila dynasty. They don't know any kind of retreat at the battle ground. If white blood cells become tired of fighting against venom, we can consider the retreat of white blood cells from the front to the back and send strong cells in waiting to the front battle ground by the strategic plan. The reality is no retreat at all and fights until they die. There is no difference in concept, only different words between oriental and modern medicines.

Now I will introduce how to solve the itching. Try to stab three to four times on the mosquito bite with a lancet needle as soon as the mosquito stings on the body skin. The lancet needle is a needle to poke the tip of a finger to check sugar level. This is a disposable needle. You may use the needle after sterilizing. Upon pricking mosquito venom and a part of white blood cells will soak out. You may feel itching a little bit, but this itching will be disappeared soon. As the venom comes into the body, taking out the venom out of the body is the best way. One time is enough on most cases, but itching comes back sometimes on the next day. You can do the above described procedure again.

It is the best to do the above procedure immediately right after the mosquito bite, but there is a time we can't take any emergency action. The bitten area becomes very large in severe cases. We use the suction cup to remove the venom. The blood drawn out by the suction cup is very thick like cranberry which we eat with turkey on Thanksgiving Day. Unless this bad blood is not taken out, the blood may circulate the body and block the capillaries in the head causing cerebral infarction. Do you think only cholesterol to block the capillaries? The answer is no.

I heard Bill and Melinda Foundation funded billions dollars to create a vaccine for mosquito venom. I sent a letter to the foundation saying I have some ideas to save a lot of money replacing the vaccine. I got a reply saying they do not accept the individual idea, but only from the corporation. How much does it cost to buy a few lancet needles to native people in Africa or where lots of mosquitos are dominated? How much does it cost to educate the above described information? I believe the remained fund can be used for other project, but this money doesn't belong to me anyhow, and the owner may do whatever he wants for better purposes.

You can watch You-Tube how to use the suction cup.

https://www.youtube.com/watch?v=28aykvUgkwM

BEE STING

Even though I did take an action I didn't get good results for bee sting. I suspect the bee poison may be able to spread very easily beyond the defense line of the body. My body was covered with rashes like soap bubbles after a bee sting and looked awesome. I heard these rashes reach and cover the neck making the person to die due to difficult breathing. Thank, God, it didn't happen to me.

The best way is to take anti-histamine from the pharmacy. The next thing is to use the suction cup and extract the blood and bee poison. Even though you do this, the poisoned area is swollen, itching and fever with red skin color. If you can buy bo-he(mint) leaves, apply these leaves without stems unto the area and cover with the bandage. Febrifuge function in Bo-he leaves will mitigate throbbing pain significantly.

I heard every year someone die with bee sting while cutting the grass of the grave around Chusuk (Korean Thanksgiving). I suggest bringing antihistamine in advance. This may prevent deaths due to bee sting. Drinking alcohol should not be allowed for this bee sting.

ORGAN DONATION

The development of medical technology saves the lives of many people. One of them is the organ transplant surgery. Something that can't imagine in the past is becoming a reality. The development of anatomy can make many kinds of surgeries possible. The surgery of liver and kidney is almost generalized and the heart transplant surgery is often done.

Many people want to live longer. This hope becomes possible with the development of medical technology. One of the ways is by organ transplants. However the demand is a lot more than the supply in the reality.

Some religious groups do the campaign to participate this movement to save many dying people. The ultimate purpose of the religion is to love each other. When I die, I donate my organs that are not anymore useful to someone and save the precious life. How wonderful idea it is!

Before I continue the story, I am an acupuncturist and believe the theory of oriental medicines. For example the kidney governs the hair on the head according to oriental theory. One patient gave me a story that a 79 years old man with gray hairs got the kidney transplant from a 29years old man. Since then this old man got black hairs. Modern science proves the theory of oriental medicine.

CELLULAR MEMORY

There are a lot of unexpected things happened after a heart transplant. These stories are published by the book and mentioned a lot through the media.

1. One man has had a nightmare every night after the heart transplant. Someone tries to kill him. As these nightmares continued every night, he was scared of becoming the night. He found the heart was transplanted by the man who was murdered. His nightmare was the moment to be murdered. He sketched the murder's picture and submitted it to the police station. The police were able to arrest the killer. This is contrary to a belief of western medicine that the heart has a function only to pump the blood from veins to arteries.

2. One old man got the artificial heart transplant as he couldn't wait for the human beings heart. Since then he had no problem to live, but unexpected issues occurred. This man had grandchildren. He knew to love grandchildren by brain, but had no desire to love by heart. As the artificial heart has no emotion to love, this may be a natural result. When we are asked once in while where the mind is, we usually point the chest instead of head. We unconsciously know the mind resided at the heart as the oriental medicine interprets.

3. One country girl's personality has changed since the heart transplant. She used to love the classical music and have the quiet personality. After the surgery she loves pro wrestling and rock music. While she watches pro wrestling games one player throws other player at the mat, she yells just like a rolling house. If her parents ask her why you do something you have never done, she talks back "What are you talking about?" and becomes rebellious. As parents believe all these happen after the heart transplant, they go to the hospital and discuss. They ask whose heart. This information is confidential, so cannot be given according to the hospital. However parents finally found the address of the donor and went to the address. The donor was a truck driver. He was killed during the driving. As he signed the anatomical gift on his driver license, his organs distributed

to a few hospitals. His parents also testified he loved the pro wrestling and rock music while he was alive.

4. One man is a macho type of guy who love screaming and hanging out with his friends. After he got the female heart for the heart transplant, he became to love cooking, cleaning, house decoration and even knitting. His wife is very happy about his change, but he is planning to sue the hospital as the hospital didn't mention about the female heart.

5. The most recent news is the business man in the 60s. He likes sports after the heart transplant. He attended various games and received trophies and certificates of winning and proudly displayed them in the living room. He also cried over listening to a radio while driving with his wife. His wife and friends puzzled these matters and looked for the reason. Their finding was the heart came from a stunt man. Who is the stuntman? Stuntmen usually do the good exercise and do the dangerous action instead of actors to prevent actors hurt. His friends also testified that he loves one female singer and moved to tears while listening to her song.

6. Most heart receivers feel the heart now is not his own. They feel the heart says this is not the right place that the heart resides and wants to get out.

I know more stories like these examples. Not only regular function of the heart by western medicine, but also the spirit is stored in the heart by oriental medicine. Oriental medicine also defines other organs do the similar features.

DEFINITION OF THE SPIRIT IN ORIENTAL MEDICINE

Heart: spirit, Lungs: departing soul, liver: soul, spleen: will, wisdom, kidney: intention, essence

Surgeries on liver and kidney are done very often and any abnormal things are not shown on the most cases after the surgery. However the heart shows many examples as described above. I believe this happens as the spirit resides at the heart. I interpret soul and departing soul as a shadow of the spirit, therefore they don't appear greatly. Will, wisdom, intention and essence don't appear greatly, neither.

The spirit of heart is different. Another spirit comes into the body and exists together. We may not have to do the heart transplant to prolong the life under the good name of science. Christianity teaching is to love others with the body and soul. These teaching and science combined may hide the Satan's master minded deception of organ donations.

WORLD OF IMAGINATION

Let me ask a question. Christians believe in the resurrection and rapture. The rapture means to be lifted as its current state. Mr. A donates all organs including eyes and nose to Mr. B and dies. When Jesus comes to judge the world, whom do these donated organs belong to? Before you answer almighty God will take care of that, the Bible says this way.

Jesus said Thomas who doubted the resurrection to check marks of the nail on palms and the side. Jesus was resurrected with most glorious moments. He didn't get the plastic surgery for the beauty. If Mr. B doesn't want to give back from the above example as Mr. A donated to Mr. B voluntarily, whose organs will Mr. A get? If Mr. A has a notorious life, this donation maybe the most glorious moment of his life.

Even though some Christians believe this donation is a good decision, will this person live without eyes and nose in the heaven? The judgment is yours. It may be quite natural for this person to be treated like that in the heaven as he had a notorious life. But if this man lived a good life based on faith, the story is complicated.

There is no one to describe the kingdom of heaven in detail. Please judge this question according to your faith and knowledge.

Please consider also this reality. Some are born with a weak heart, or deaf. Some are born blind as mentioned in the Bible.

Let us assume someone lost his life due to black market trafficking. If he claims that I didn't give the organ voluntarily and give back to him, what is the judgment of God?

I recall the philosophy class in the university. The professor told this story. I try to tell you exactly literally, so don't consider the religious color. Two friends passed by and killed by the thieves in the desert. One wife heard about this news and went to the scene. She found two necks and bodies separated. She prayed "Almighty God, help me." and picked up heads and attached necks to bodies. The dead bodies become alive. The problem is she did this hastily, and she found the head is her husband and the body is his friend's. Which one must she choose the head or the body? If she chooses the head, it is metaphysical. If she chooses the body, it is physical according to the professor.

It may be not far off that the story as fancy as the above story will be a reality.

If the carotid was cut in the past, we must die. But due to the good world the surgery may make to revive now. Let us assume someone commits a crime and exchanges his head with other person. Witness testifies obviously the face, but the perpetrator through the police investigation concludes the body as the finger prints belong to the body. Whom are you going to punish? This kind of scenario would be a problem in this world. Let me ask another question. How does this person when they resurrect?

Personal opinion

1. Man gets from another man's heart and woman gets from another woman's. I believe this is the principle for the heart transplant.

2. The personality may be similar with the constitution according to ideology of oriental medicine. I believe if western medicine applies this theory into the heart transplant; the usual side effects of different personality would be less.

3. I am going to refuse to receive organs of any other people, but not to give either. Please don't throw a stone for my faith. Old saying is we receive even hairs and skin from parents, therefore not to undermine them is the beginning of the filial piety for parents. I believe this is the wisdom of the old adults.

All transplants surgeries are done by thinking only of function of organs without considering the spiritual world. But if the principles of the oriental medicine are right, we can't claim all transplant surgeries are right as a lot of unexplainable things are happening. This is the reason we need careful discussion now.

Why Women live longer than men

All statistics report that women live longer than men. Average age of men is 75.74 and women's age is 82.36years old. Women live 6.62 years longer. In the past the difference was more than 8 years, but now the number is gradually declining. However there still is no change that women live longer than men. Why does this happen?

I heard a pastor's sermon that the material is different with men and women. While God creates Adam with soils, God creates Eve using Adam's rib. So as bones are much more durable than the clay, women live longer than men.

Male sex hormones

The male sex hormone is generated during the puberty. The sudden change in the body makes them difficult to control, leads to violence in the worst case.

Man has stress more likely

As men are responsible for the survival of the home, they have greater stress from the outside. Women's stress is confined to the home, but men are engaged in more complicated and difficult tasks from the outside.

Different methods to reduce the stress

Anyone will be exposed to the stress. Stress may be better or worse depending on the type how constructive it is. The way is a little bit different to relieve the bad stress between men and women. Women have a tendency to chat with friends, but men engage in rather alcohol and tobacco to relieve the stress. Women are constructive and men are destructive. The quantity of alcohol and tobacco is also great.

THE FREQUENCY SEEKING THE HOSPITAL

The man is taught and raised to be strong since the kid. We teach not to cry even on stumbling. The man doesn't like to show the weakness to others. This kind of nature makes men to be reluctant to go to the hospital. There are a lot more women than men who come to our clinic. This means any diseases can be found, treated and prevented earlier for women.

VIOLENT BEHAVIOR

Men do the more radical than women. Even in fighting women fight with words and pull hair each other in the severe case. But for men the baseball bat is a basic tool. The dangerous stuff like a knife is used to wound or even kill. Women drive modestly, but men drive recklessly making other people scary. These factors are to be believed in a valid reason making a man hasten the life.

These reasons are generally accepted and true and have valid reasons, but don't look like a whole picture.

THE VIEW FROM ORIENTAL MEDICINE

I mentioned already that the man belongs to yang and the woman belongs to yin. There are also yin and yang in the organs. Some organs belong to yang and other organs belong to yin. The organs which belong to yin are liver, heart, spleen, lungs and kidneys. Yang organs are gallbladder, small intestine, stomach, large intestine and urinary bladder. The important thing to remember is yin organs keep moving all the time. Yang organs work only when needed and take a break. If a person is not breathing through lungs, this means an emergency for the life. The heart also works always. However the stomach works only while foods are in the stomach. If there is no food, the stomach takes a break. Small intestine and large intestine do the same way.

The principle of organs also applies to human beings. Men work hard while working. But when the work is over, men try to forget all things. When the husband returns home in the past, he asks his wife to bring water. Even though he can do this by himself, he orders his wife. He then sits on the sofa and reads the newspaper without lifting a finger or turns on TV. Many people will nod and agree. In fact this is the principle. When women listen to this, they may not be able to agree at all. However this is the story of the past. The present situation is the husband cannot breathe over the power of wife. I believe this current situation also contributes the shortage of life.

But women do work all little things restlessly all days. After cooking she washes dishes. At the end of washing dishes, she cleans the rooms. After cleaning she waters plants. Oh I forgot the laundries. When she tries to have her own time alone, children come back home. Another war will start.

Let us assume this family lives in this way until the retirement. The problem occurs when the man retires. Women constantly move as usual. Men were at peaks while men make money, but now the situation is changed. His position is shabby and ragged. Men have a plan to have a trip which has been postponed for a life. Right after the trip his lifetime goal is achieved and leads for the loss of goals for the future. This loss of goals and the position of the back burner will affect the life expectancy.

After the retirement a man opens eyes in the morning habitually. He realizes he doesn't have to get up now as he retired and stay in the bed. When this situation is repeated, the cell that wakes him up in the morning gradually becomes to weaken and destroyed eventually. Cells to remember the time to go to work and ride on the subway will be forgotten gradually. Therefore the man must plan the post-retirement ahead and do not make this kind of stupid things. It must be a good idea to do some volunteering work or do some gardening in the back yard.

Cultural life changed

However the current life is much different from the past. A lot of men push and ask wives to make money and many women join for the employment. The social distinction between men and women increasingly becomes obsolescent. As the activity of women increases, the role in the house has changed accordingly. Many men begin and participate in the household chores and childcare. I believe this kind of reality reduces the difference between male and female life.

The pursuit of the beauty

Women consider the beauty more important than men. Other parts of the body can be covered, but not with the face and head. Therefore women invest heavily on the face and head, so frequent touches are followed. Not only just washing the face with a soap, but also wipe the face off with cleansing and nutrition cream. What about brushing hair? The better blood circulation will follow naturally on the face and head. Bone marrows are stored a lot in the brain and these movement described invigorate the bone marrow vigorously.

There is an exception that the woman wakes up with lion's hair and takes care of families.

Physiological differences

Female

No matter how the society changes, there is no change that the woman is pregnant and gives a birth. The woman does the menstruation. If the pregnancy doesn't occur, the woman has a marvelous structure to discharge the egg as well as the blood stasis. The blood stasis means blood clots. The blood stasis causes a disturbance in the blood circulation. The new blood is produced replacing the blood clots. However the man doesn't have this feature. I believe this kind of woman's structure affects greatly to live a longer life.

Another factor is the man can be ready to ejaculate not only for the pregnancy but also the physiological response anytime and anywhere, but the woman prepares the egg only once a month in operation. So the frequency is another matter.

MALE

Old books recommend the man not to use the semen for nothing. When the man preserves the essence (semen) like a treasure, this is enabling for the man to live longer. The books emphasize the importance of the essence. The man emits the semen out physiologically. The woman does once a month, but the man can emit without much efforts meaning a lot more frequency. When the man drunk, the erection becomes easy temporally and the emission is followed.

While young this happens often and eventually affects the man's life.

The article that eunuchs lived longer than the ordinary people supports the above theory. Who is the eunuch? The person is castrated while a kid. It is impossible for the emission of sperm and semen.

I believe priests and monks who don't do the sex life may live longer than ordinary people.

FOUR CONSTITUTIONS

Four constitutions is the oriental medicine theory of Lee Jema many people are aware of to the public in Korea. There are taiyang, shaoyin, shaoyang and taiyin as most people understand.

Some patients occasionally ask a question what the constitution is for them. The reason is simple. When anyone tries analysis for his own constitution through the newspaper or the magazine, it is not easy to determine. They feel that he or she belongs to this constitution or that constitution. So they want to find out the sure one as they come to the clinic.

This request is the reasonable one. Some patients complain that A clinic advised this type (taiyang) and other clinic advised that type (shaoyang). Is that possible for one person to have two different constitutions? Does the constitution change on each time or each clinic? Why does this happen? Is any other way to tell?

YIN AND YANG

When the sun shines on the hill, one side becomes the sunny spot and the opposite side becomes the shaded lot. But when the sunny spot is in the morning, it changes into the shaded spot in the afternoon. Yin changes into yang, and yang changes into yin. Yin and yang is the beginning point in the oriental medicine.

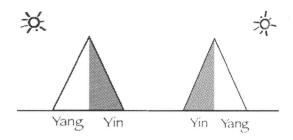

NO ABSOLUTE IN YIN AND YANG

There is another theory that there is no absolute. This means there is no total yin or total yang. For example here is a magnet. One side points to north and the other side points to south. If you cut the magnet in halves, there must be a neutral point theoretically. But this never happens. These two smaller magnets point north and south again. This means the small portion of north exits in the south side and the small portion of south exits in the north in the conclusion. Yin and yang act on the same principle.

We often see the unique figure in Aikido or self-defense practicing room. This figure represents the yin and yang.

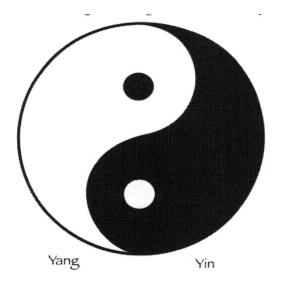

Yang   Yin

The upper part is yang and the lower part is yin. The left side is yang and the right side is yin. The point in the middle displays the conception. The right moment of the absolute means the beginning of the opposite.

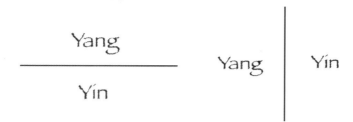

There are yin and yang in Pic 1. When we divide yin in half, there are two parts of yin and yang. When we also divide yang in half, there are also two parts of yin and yang. Let us divide into four as follows.

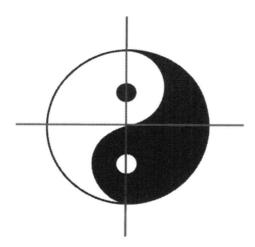

If we describe in different ways, the picture of yin and yang is divided into good four. If we center horizontally, the upper side is yang and the lower side is yin. If we center vertically, the left side is yang and the right side is yin. The bottom left is yin and yang (-. +), the upper left is yang and yang (+,+), the upper right is yang and yin (+,-) and the lower right is yin and yin (-,-). (Pic 5)

Therefore the bottom left is shaoyin, the upper left is taiyang, the upper right is shaoyang and the lower right is taiyin.

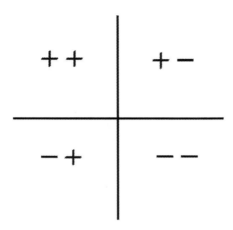

The large part of yin is taiyin and the other small part is shaoyang. When we divide yang, there are also two parts of yin and yang. The large part of yang is taiyang and the other small part of is shaoyin. (Pic 6)

Tai Yang	Shao Yang
Shao Yin	Tai Yin

SUMMER	FALL
SPRING	WINTER

RELATIONSHIP BETWEEN SEASONS AND CONSTITUTIONS

This becomes spring, summer, autumn and winter in the season. When we combine the above, these become spring=shaoyin, summer=taiyang, fall=shaoyang, and winter=taiyin. Therefore the person born in the spring is spring constitution, in summer is summer constitution, in fall is fall constitution and in winter is winter constitution. In other words the person born in spring is shaoyin, in summer is taiyang, in fall is shaoyang and in winter is taiyin. Everyone knows the date of birth. This is the four constitutions theory. Is this difficult? The original oriental medicine is not to memorize, rather to understand the law of nature

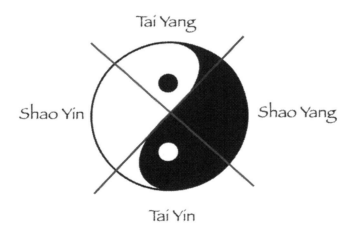

YIN & YANG AND CONSTITUTIONS

But there are two problems. The first thing is as I mentioned already, the oriental theory is based on yin and yang and the five elements.

We have to add the late summer into spring, summer, fall and winter. You already understand seasons. The summer is usually hot and relatively less rain. A rainy season is followed in the late summer. Typhoons are in Asia and hurricanes are in America. It is also a season that more damp prevail. This is the reason many people confuse which constitutions belong to due to only four constitutions. Therefore classifications into five constitutions are close to the theory of oriental medicine.

The second question is when the spring begins and ends. There are differences of the season between we feel and the universe moves. For example the first day of the spring (ground hog day) according to the lunar calendar is about third on February, but it is cold enough for us to have to wear a coat. It is usually one month later when we actually feel the spring.

This is spring constitution and belongs to shaoyin according to four constitutions. However I classify five constitutions, so I try to name it by season.

(This illustration is from the book of "5 seasons, 5 constitutions in health)

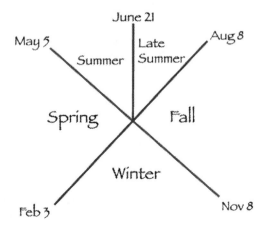

Spring constitution: February 3-May 5(the beginning day of summer)

Summer constitution: May5-June 21(summer solstice)

Late summer constitution: June 21-August 8(the beginning day of fall)

Fall constitution: August 8-November 8(the beginning day of winter)

Winter constitution: November 8-February 3(the beginning of spring)

The exact date may be slightly different every year.

The next question is to eat what foods are good for the body. Spring constitution eats 20% more foods produced in the spring than other foods. These are barley, shepherd's purse, dandelion and wild green vegetables in the spring. It is relatively easy to tell for summer, late summer and fall. It is the food produced by the season. You may use seafood for winter.

Hair Loss

The hair loss between men and women are different. The hair loss for men occurs in a specific part of the head, but for women occurs lightly as a whole. Western medicine explains it due to the influence of hormones. Oriental medicine describes it caused by the heat.

Oriental medicine starts from yin and yang in everything. Men belong to yang and women belong to yin. Warmth belongs to yang and cold belongs to yin. Men have generally warm body and women have cold body. Of course this is different individually, but this theory can be applied in overall.

The next problem is the difference between yin and yang. It depends on which one is larger, yin and yang.

Root cause of Hair loss

The root cause of hair fall is due to the drying of the hair follicle.

For example weeds in summer are very strong. The weed grows between concrete blocks in my house. I try to take it out, so I hold it tight by hand. Main roots grow deep down in order to draw water and nutrients. Many small roots do the same thing from the main roots. All these roots hold tight under the ground. I pluck it out with all my strength, and removed only leaves and some stems and a portion of the top, but the root remained the same. So I gave up and waited the summer is over. In the fall, I hold the bottom of the weed and fixed firmly my feet on the ground and pulled out with all my strength. My body fell over backward. The reason is simple. I didn't consider the less holding power, which is cohesion of the weed, so I gave more power than needed while I was thinking the past experience.

Some say they find many hairs on the pillow after sleeping or shampooing from the shower. Some complain hair falling by just combing. It is the same theory for the weeds and hairs. Hairs will be fallen off with dry follicles holding the hair.

REASON OF DRY FOLLICLE

The reason of dry follicle is due to low-grade fever. The fever evaporates the moisture, and then the dryness follows. The water is required to get rid of the fever. Oriental medicine believes this is done by kidneys. The kidneys have two functions: making water (kidney yin) and lifting water (kidney yang). Selection of acupuncture points is important as well as the depth of needles in my opinion. Master Hur Im also believed that the depth of needles influences greatly. The author Hur Jun of Eastern Oriental medicine treasure recognized that Hur Im is the master as far as acupuncture is concerned.

Of course the effectiveness would be great with herbal medicines. Scalp massage or drugs on head can provide transient effective, but can't be fundamental root treatments. Therefore time and money can be saved with oriental medicine. The reason is not only to treat symptoms but also the root cause.

DIFFERENT TYPES OF HAIR LOSS AGAINST MALE

There are several types of hair loss in men: alopecia hair loss of the front part and vertex part of the head. There are coin size, football size, highway type and English M-type in more details of alopecia.

I personally believe the hair loss from the front part may be acceptable, but the vertex area may be not that good. The front part of hair loss is due to too much stamina. As the husband wants too often and long for the sex, his wife pushes his forehead by her hand asking him stop. But the hair loss at the vertex is due to the different reason. As the man is a patient of premature ejaculation, his wife holds his head asking stay longer. Please don't take it seriously as this is a joke.

Everyone has cold and warm at the same time. But the women have more warmness on the upper body and more coldness in the lower body. The rate of hair loss of women is less than men as men have more heat than women.

EXCESSIVE HEAT AND EMPTY HEAT

The following explanation may be a little difficult to understand for the ordinary person. These are excessive heat and empty heat. The perfect condition is 100 each in yin and yang. It is almost impossible and difficult to achieve or maintain this status for anyone.

If the yin is 100 and the yang is 120, the yang is higher than the yin by 20. The body tries to eliminate this excessive 20 to make a balance. This amount of 20 is the excessive heat.

In contrast the yin is 60 and the yang is 90. The oriental medicine calls this status Yin deficiency. 90 is less than perfect, but the body feels fever, so this is not the true heat, that's why we call this as the empty heat. In this situation the body tries to make the balance by eliminating the difference of 30. Many women have been experienced the night sweating during the menopause meaning when getting up, sweating in the whole body. This is due to the empty heat.

Another method is to fill this deficiency of 30. However this deficiency is not filled on time, the empty heat rises and stays to the head. The hair loss begins due to the empty heat and number of hairs will be diminished. This will make yin and yang in balance ultimately, but the aging would be developed further causing wrinkles, osteoporosis and depression and other bad influences. So the best way is to fill the deficiency yin, 30.

This is just one reference. This case is the yin is 90 while the yang is 60. The yin has the nature of cold, so this person may always feel cold. I sometimes heard "I have been cold all my life, but now even though I do have another health issues, but I am not cold as used to be." This means the yin becomes 70 or 60 or even 50.

The treatment method is for men to get rid of the excessive heat and for women to fill the yin deficiency in general. Don't think of only hair loss alone as all organs are interrelated. Do not think all people do suffer this way while experiencing menopause. Please confront this status more actively.

But the Eastern oriental medicine treasure interprets another way. As hairs grow upwards, hairs on head belong to the heart. Eyebrows that grow sideways belong to the liver. As the beard grows downward, the beard belongs to the kidney. This is really plausible theory. Can we say old ancients are less intelligent than moderns? I never thought about this theory, but ancients already observed and wrote this incredible theory.

This is the experience when I went to the Amazon River. After getting off from the boat and walked for a while, the Indians came to meet us. I couldn't see the breast directly, but were able to see from the side as they covered the breast with a small mat weaved with reeds. Female Indians asked me to dance. The breast of young girls has a large volume. While my partner danced with me, she moved back and forth. I had to watch her with my head to the side. I saw her breast. The breast looked like a sagging one of a very old woman. But her hairs were black. I asked the travel guide how she has black hairs even though she looks old. She answered she washed her hairs with her urine. This way prevents hair loss and does not need to have her hair dyed. Would you try by yourself?

Some men eat frogs and snakes for more stamina. Some women do the plastic surgery for the beauty these days. Is it worth with washing hairs with urine to prevent the hair loss?

This is a joke, but I have thought this idea for a long time. My first thought was this may be related with oxygen as the Amazon River provides more than 50% of oxygen amount of the world. I finally reached to this conclusion. This may be due to salts in the urine. So I washed my hair with salt water instead of pee. Salts are contended in our body. When the high concentration of salt is present upon the human body, the osmotic pressure will act on the skin. This osmosis makes the blood move to the outer skin and provides nutrients to the scalp.

Try to use a shampoo with mint ingredients. The mint has a function to eliminate the heat.

Of course the best way is to get acupuncture and herbal treatments. As you understand now, these are able to treat the root cause.

HYPERTENSION AND SALT

We heard so many recommendations of doctors not to smoke and take too much salts. Does eating salty really induce the hypertension? I don't think so. I try to think about the relationship between salt and hypertension hard, but I couldn't find a good reason without one.

When you eat much salt, we have to drink more water naturally. This is the natural body reaction. Our body tries to retain more water in order to maintain the proper concentration of the salt amount. The retained water flows through the blood vessels and the concentration level becomes back to normal, then the retained water will be discharged. Modern sciences worry if the extra water is accumulated, the heart is supposed to work hard to send the extra accumulated water, so the blood pressure goes up. Do you agree? I don't think so.

1. This may be a little difficult to understand, so read this carefully. The heart is similar with a pump receiving from one side to sending out the other side. The heart receives the blood from the veins and sends to other organs to exchange oxygen from carbon dioxide and discharges to arteries. The reason of high blood pressure is due to the increasing velocity in order to send a large amount of blood through the small cross-sectional area. But if the small cross-sectional area becomes larger, the velocity will be slowed down and the pressure will also be decreased. If we eat the salty foods, the blood volume increases. This will also increase the cross-section area. This will lead to decrease the velocity and also the pressure. Someone may claim the blood vessels of the arteries can't be stretched. This may be right on the condition of coronary infarction. However the blood vessels of healthy person should be increased in my opinion. I intentionally had salty. The

weight was two pounds more than normal. I also tried to eat one whole box of ice cream. This also increased two pounds. I drank hard liquor, too. The same 2 pounds increased. My weight is 150 pounds, so only 1.3% increase. There is no difference between salt and sugar. I believe our heart may be able to tolerate enough to hold even 5%.

If we mark this as a symbol, it is as follows.
Quantity = (AREA) x (VELOCITY)
Q= total amount of blood
A= section of diameter of blood vessel
V= speed of blood passing the above section
(Total blood amount in vein)= (Total blood amount in artery)
$q1 = q2$
We can say now
$q1 = a1 \times v1, q2 = a2 \times v2$

An artery is a smaller blood vessel surrounded by thick muscle located deep inside of body. This artery vessel is difficult to expand, whereas a vein is easy to expand, as the vein is thin and located around a superficial area.

Therefore, as a2 is smaller than a1, v2 is faster than v1. As v1 is slow in flowing, any deposits are easy to settle in a1 which is in vein. The deposits in artery are relatively difficult as the velocity is faster in artery. Of course, all deposits begin from vein. When there is only a little room left in the vein, deposits starts to accumulate in the artery. When the person has a chest pain and a diagnosis of an artery blockage in the heart, more than 70-75% of that section of the blood vessel is already blocked. It is wrong to wait until 70-75% of a blood vessel is blocked. Then there is not much choice except surgery. It might require a number of surgeries as there could be more blockages.

2. Before the refrigerator had been used like nowadays, we used to marinate foods to prevent spoilage. For example there are pickled shrimp, or cod roe which are very salty. I

believe these foods are consumed in the winter time. How many years do refrigerators be generalized? It was less than 60 years. Do you think our DNA is able to adapt within 60 years? DNA has been built over more than a few thousand years. Modern medicines are about 100 years, but I don't believe DNA will be changed in a few years.

3. Please refer the next column of five tastes. Salt water in the sea raises the vaporization at 26 degree Celsius. Therefore eating salty foods in the winter time would be in effects for warmth. We can apply this that who has cold body in nature could make body warm by eating a little more salty foods. Of course who has a warm body should take more bitter tastes foods.

4. All animals accumulate the salt in order to prevent the decay. I mentioned already fishes in freshwater are tasted better for spicy soup and fishes in saltwater are better for sushi with sour and hot paste. When we ask the reason to eat salty, the answer tastes better. Oriental medicine defines the deficiency of spleen function causes less appetite. The spleen deficiency will cause phlegm. Salt eventually helps the function of the spleen. The salt also features the ability to prevent spoilage. Foot necrosis may follow in severe diabetes. We may explain in different ways. One theory is when the sugar content is increased; the capillaries become sticky and end up being blocked causing necrosis.

5. Then how can we prevent necrosis? More water can dilute the sticky, doesn't it? It is difficult to force drinking water, but salty eating makes a lot easy to drink more water.

6. Cancer can grow anywhere except finger and toe nails and hairs. Most people do not hear the heart cancer. Why? The reason is the heart contains more salts. Koreans call the heart with a special name; salt container. The heart has to move continuously without a break. No moving means the death. The heart must be soft instead of hard.

How can be soft? Have you ever seen to prepare Korean Kim chi? It looks like a mountain of Chinese cabbages in the beginning. Salted water is added into them and waits for the next day. The volume of them becomes a lot smaller on the next day as they become very soft. One of medicines of western medicines for the blood pressure pills is the calcium-channel blocker. This is to prevent the heart hardening. My question is why not to take much salt and prescribe the blocker.

7. We know kidneys are organs to take care of water. Kidneys must also have a little more salt content to discharge water. This will create the osmotic effects to bring water into kidneys easy. Advising to take less salt without taking into this kind of account does not fit the principle.

8. A. Oriental medicine uses some special terminology which means water climbing up and fire going down. This concept is contrary to the common sense. However if a fire just goes up and can't come down in the human body, the head becomes hot, but the feet become cold. The heat must be distributed evenly on the entire body to maintain the healthy body, otherwise we may become sick. Therefore the cold water goes up and cools down the heat. It is just like the boiling water in the pot. Then how can the cold water be raised up by oriental theory? This is the role of salt. Everyone knows it is easy for swimming in the ocean than the river.

   B. I make a fruit juice in the morning. I make slices from fruits and place the chopped fruits in a blender with water. When I add bamboo salt into the water, sliced fruits float up.

   C. This is another example. How do clouds be made? The hot sun shines on the ocean. Ocean water doesn't boil, but changes into vapor and goes up into the sky. The reason happen more in the ocean rather than in the river is that the ocean contains in the ocean rather than in the river is that the ocean contains more salt.

9. The whole issue is the quality of salt not on over consumption of the salt. Most of us use cheap salt rather than the sea salt. This is the problem. Cheap salt contains sodium only, but no necessary minerals. Human body has sympathetic and parasympathetic nerves. Sympathetic nerves are related with sodium chloride and parasympathetic nerves are with potassium. While cheap salt is used, sympathetic nerves act excessively, but parasympathetic nerves cannot act properly due to lack of necessary minerals. This means the unbalance between yin and yang.

10. Even western medicine study does not comply with this theory that salty eating increase the hypertension. Why does this happen? There are two possibilities.

Q=(AREA) x (VELOCITY)

If Q is increased and Area also is increased, velocity remains the same as the elasticity of blood vessel is normal. But if hardening of blood vessel happens, the blood vessel can't be expended. Then velocity would be increased and the pressure is also increased.

Some studies show that if there is no eating salt, the hormone production would stop.

11. Even natural sea salt contains pollution as all the pollutants in the earth reach to the sea. So we need the salt which doesn't contain pollutants. There is only one product in Korea called Bamboo salt. Regular sea salts are packed into the bamboos. Heat the bamboos on 1000 degree Celsius. While burning bamboos, most pollutants are burned too. Some products repeat this process nine times, so very expensive. I personally use twice baked bamboo salt, as the

PH concentration of this salt is about 7.2 which is the most ideal concentration for the human body.

12. When diuretic is the first commercially available, the symptoms of hypertension may be over forever. They believe high blood pressure may be resolved by the incremental emissions as the hypertension is caused due to increased blood amount than normal. Actually there were many effects from diuretic use. But over time, problems start to occur. Kidney realizes more water come into and less blood than required. Kidney requests the brain to send more blood into the kidney and the brain gives a signal and makes the heart to pump more blood. Something never expected has happened. The scientists develop a prescription drug that suppressed the signal. This may control blood pressure, but kidney function becomes worse. Why don't send more blood necessary than inhibiter?

Quantity = (AREA) x (VELOCITY)

The diuretic is the function for reducing Quantity. As quantity is reduced, the pressure would be reduced due to the reducing velocity even though area is not changed. My personal opinion is for determining the amount of diuretic is not easy. The problem is the density of the blood would be thicker than normal by the diuretic. I believe more thrombus would be produced. In order to avoid this, the blood thinner is used which may be artificial and chemical. The other side effects of diuretic are not in my professional, so ask professionals.

13. Without considering this fact, just blood thinner is prescribed. I believe it is more desirable to consider all the related organs instead of just symptoms. Many patients may take medicines without knowing this fact. Many patients believe they have to take high blood pressure pills until they die. This is a big mistake just like a young elephant. Do you know how to train young elephants? When elephant is

young, trainers place young elephant to tie into the sturdy rope hung on the ground. Young elephant realizes no matter how much he tries and cannot move. Even though these elephants grow by huge enough to move very strong stake, they just give up moving when they see just a piece of rope. A lot of patients with hypertension believe they should take medicines for a lifetime just like being tied to the frame. This is not an exaggeration.

Many patients experience becoming better with acupuncture and herb treatments. The reason is due to the unique concept of heart and kidney meaning fire and water. This will treat original causes as well as symptoms. Now all you have to lower the amount of pills gradually based on situation with discussion with your MD who prescribe for you.

FIVE TASTES AND FIVE COLORS

The tongue distinguishes sour, bitter, sweet, spicy and salty. My conclusion from these is to take all these five tastes. However most people take their favorites foods only, and don't take their dislike foods. For example people like sweet, spicy and salty and don't like sour and bitter.

When someone gets the benefit of sour taste, they become a mania of the sour taste. The body feels so great with that. This person sometimes asks the friend or closed one to drink vinegar; however most of them make frowned face asking how possible to drink the sour vinegar. She drinks this vinegar water made by brown rice a few times a day. There was a time citric acid had been popular. This is the one that has sour taste.

One thing common is most don't like bitter taste except who drink black coffee only. I used to joke this story often. The reason why herbal medicine is bitter is due to the supplementary of bitterness as the patient has not taken enough bitter taste foods. I don't drink coffee personally, but I don't oppose drinking coffee greatly. The reason is most people don't take bitter taste foods except drinking coffee. Drinking coffee may be an only source to take bitter taste.

I repeat to remind you if you stress only one side causing a disease. Therefore we have to take foods of all tastes: only one or two tastes will cause a disease.

YELLOW EMPEROR'S INNER CANON AND ORIENT MEDICINE TREASURE

These books are the oldest in the oriental medicine. These books explain about five tastes. I try to use this application, but it was difficult to understand. I try to figure the formula and give up. I looked another books, but the result is the same. I have contemplated this principle and obesity for a long time and may find some relationship. A famous pastor often says "even though my opinion is not always right". I try to apply this word here. Here is a table for the general purpose.

Spring	Summer	Late summer	Fall	Winter
Liver	Heart	Spleen	Lung	Kidney
Sour	Bitter	Sweet	Spicy	salty

Spring and summer are seasons for energy to climb up. Fall and winter are to go down. The energy climbs up a little in the spring and rises more in the summer. The energy goes down a little in the fall and more in the winter.

While the energy is climbing up, the holding energy comes from sour taste. As the energy belongs to yang, the taste belongs to yin. The holding sour energy makes a balance against the rising energy.

It is very hot in the summer. It is the season when the energy is very strong. We can interpret this energy means a lot of heat. The heart is supposed to send lots of heat. What is going to happen if the heat goes up and can't come down? Many symptoms will follow headache as well as high blood pressure, red face and losing consciousness. Therefore the bitter taste has the role of lowering heat down.

Let me give you some information about the bitter taste. Western medicine thinks the bile is made by the combination of red blood cells destructed and cholesterol. Part of the bile is used for digestion and reused with reabsorption. While the diarrhea is going on, the body couldn't absorb.

I'd like to explain the formation of the bile this way. The bile is extremely bitter. Everyone knows the bear bile is very bitter. Many experience even the very small amount of the bear bile with mixed wine. Why is it so bitter?

When we eat bitter foods, our body absorbs the bitter and concentrates and stores in the gallbladder. If we don't take the bitter taste foods, we don't have raw materials for the formation of the bile. What happens on the lack of bile? When we take the fatty foods, the bile comes out to help the digestion for the fat. If the fat is not digested, the fat may remain as it is. This is the so-called fat in the body. This will lead to the obesity naturally. As many don't take bitter foods, how do you expect to make bile? Whenever bile needs in the digestion, the gallbladder repeats the squeeze the bile duct, the heat may be produced on the duck or gallbladder. The heat consumes the moisture and becomes dry. Any leftover bile on the duct could be trapped and turned into the stone. This stone becomes bigger and clogged causing the jaundice.

The sweet taste belongs to spleen and the spleen belongs to the earth. The sweet taste has a function to make dampness and eliminate the heat. Therefore the sweet is the enemy of obesity.

The spicy belongs to lungs and the season is the fall. As soon as the fall comes, the vigorous hot retreats and the cool temperature begins. This season is the energy comes down. Therefore the lifting energy is necessary in this case; spiciness. Many experiences hot and sweating after eating spicy foods like spicy peppers. In severe cases sticky saliva and tingling mouth will be continued even after drinking cold water. This is a good example of counteracting cycle. This is the example of lung counteracting to heart. As this example the taste does counter clock wise instead of clockwise.

The salty taste belongs to winter and the related organ is the kidney. It is the season the energy falls the most and everything hide. The sea is the representation of hiding. We know deep sea hides everything. Sea salt is rich in the sea. When the sun makes warm in the sea, vapor is created easily. When it reaches 26 degrees Celsius, water vapor is created. This is the reason typhoon or hurricane is created.

Here is another example. When it snows in the winter, snow melts on sprinkling with salt. Salt generates heat in the process of absorbing water by chemical action. This is the reason the ocean is not frozen easily due to containing a lot of salt.

The salty taste from salt has a function to raise the energy from the bottom to the top. The body temperature is 36.5 degrees which is higher than 26 degrees of the vaporization of the salt. This means lifting can happen at any time. A word of caution is there is a difference of concentration between human body and sea, so a little higher temperature may be required. This is so called water rising and fire falling by oriental medicine. But the problem is there is a tendency of rising due to excessive salt intake, but lack of action of downing. Therefore taking bitter foods is necessary as usual.

THEORY OF ENERGY AND TASTES

Oriental medicine defines energy and tastes as above. Oriental medicine theory has been established long time ago. However the study between all foods and energy & tastes is not fully supportive and there are different opinions between scholars. So it may be more difficult for the public. I recommend the easy method the public can understand better.

The answer is color-coded. Of course if there is a difference between colors and energy & tastes, energy and tastes have priority over colors.

CHROMATIC PLANTS

Red (appetite, heart); apples, cherries, strawberries, tomatoes, watermelon, peppers, radish, Las Barry, Pomegranates, grapes

Green (detoxification), green grapes, melon, kiwi, broccoli, cabbage, spinach, lettuce, zucchini, peas, soybeans, green tea, kale, collar, green peppers

White (immune support), bananas, pears, peaches, garlic, mushrooms, ginger, onions, potatoes, turnips, cauliflower, horseradish

purple, or black (depression, longevity); grapes, plums, currants, blue berries, figs, eggplant, asparagus, purple sweet potato, red-purple cabbage, brown seaweed, Kim algae

Yellow or orange (cancer prevention); tangerine, pineapple, mango, lemon, orange, carrot, paprika, pumpkin, walnuts, corn, sweet potatoes.

Is cigarette smoking really harmful?

When we turn on any Medias, health news is flooded. Even though there are many types of diseases and very complex to the ordinary person, medical doctors explain the difficult matters easy, so general audience can understand. Most emphasize the prevention is the best. One of the preventions is to stop smoking. Smoking is one cause of all diseases. Some TV ads from New York City's smoking cessation program show terrible pictures. One of pictures is someone who has a hole on the throat due to smoking.

One couple came. The wife asked me stop smoking for her husband. He has smoked more than 40 years. His asthma is so severe and even the hospital already abandoned his treatment as long as he smokes. While we discussed, I observed the patient. Even though five minutes had passed sitting on the sofa, he experienced difficult breathing and short of breath. Even in the hospital the only thing is to connect the oxygen according to the family and there is no other way. I told the husband "Sir, you may smoke a little bit." His wife was so upset upon hearing at me and complained "we came here for stop smoking. But you advised him to continue to smoke. What on earth can you say that?" I also believe she has every right to say that as this is a common sense.

I've given her an explanation after I beg her calm. I believe your husband already knew the smoking is bad. However even though he knew, it is difficult for him to stop smoking. We have to consider this fact. Your demand for him is stressful greater than his smoking cigarettes. My question to her may make her a little guilty feeling. That's why we came here for the help. There was no one in the family for his side as far as smoking concerned. I am the only one for his side and he became excited.

He met the best doctor ever and felt he would be better if he gets my treatment.

After his condition is improved, I told him not to smoke again. He answered yes; I am going to stop smoking.

THERE IS NO ABSOLUTE IN YIN AND YANG

This is hypothesis of oriental theory. Many believe smoking is absolutely bad and no benefit at all. I dare to say this is wrong. In other words, do I mean there are benefits for smoking? The answer is yes.

There are many women smoking cigarettes. When I ask them the question why you do smoking even though you know the smoking is bad, the answer comes back this way. Stop smoking leads to the obesity, therefore continues smoking without any other choices.

Yes. Cigarettes' smoking has a function of losing weight. According to TCM, smoking means a fire burning. The fire means hot. The hotness makes dry. The dryness means becoming thin.

When I browse the internet about this matter, this is already proven scientifically. Dr. Marina Picciotto who is a neurophysiology professor in Yale University School of Medicine has confirmed that nicotine absorbed into the body during cigarette smoking affects the brain feel-good central as well as the brain hypothalamus suppressing appetite through experiments on mice.

We are aware of the problem of obesity. The obesity is not trivial compared to the harmful tobacco. However there is no comparison between two risks, we emphasize the harmful tobacco only.

Cigarette smoking affects the smoker as well as non-smokers indirectly by secondhand smokes, but the obesity affects the subject person only. In this view the tobacco is much worse than the obesity. We have to consider the accurate comparison before we claim the tobacco smoking is unconditionally bad.

Here is another example. SARS swept Southeast Asia at the beginning of the year 2000. Hundreds of people had died from the disease. There was no one suffered or died through this disease in Korea. Many guess as Koreans eat spicy kimchee. One study reports there is no one in death who smokes. I don't know the exact reason, but I guess there is some SARS prevention material in the tobacco.

When I mention this subject, many questions are followed. What about the mercury? Mercury was used as medicine materials in the past. According to the Annals of Lee Dynasty, there was a discussion whether mercury must be used for the king's illness between herbalists due to the toxicity of mercury. They already knew there is a toxic potent of the mercury, but they concluded to use the right amount for a short period of time.

There are a few bad cases using mercury in the modern society. There was a time to fill the root canal with mercury in the dentistry. I had seen a patient to pay $50,000 to remove mercury as any leakage could damage the brain seriously. This is the result the modern society didn't use the already known knowledge of five hundred years ago. Anyhow as FDA of the United States banned the use of mercury, we are no longer to use the mercury as a medicinal herb.

People ask again what about poisonous mushroom is. What on earth is good? As a matter of fact, I was much distressed by this problem. Some find mushrooms in the mountain and eat. Some was hospitalized or even died due to the poison from the mushrooms. Then what is supposed to be good or beneficial with poison? Oriental medicine defines "treat the poison with a poison". Based on this theory, many studies result that poisonous mushrooms contain lots of anti-tumor therapeutics. Let us hope new anti-tumor overcome the cancer.

Chan Hur

Here is another example from the internet.

Death carrot grows in the Mediterranean region. This plant called Thapsia Garganica blooms pretty yellow flowers. Unlike its appearance this plant was avoided by shepherds due to poisonous weeds against cattle and sheep. That's why this plant is called death carrot in ancient Greek literature between shepherds. However the research has been going on more than 15 years as this toxicity has an efficacy in killing cancer cells.

Poison can be treated by poison. The day will come here soon when the use of toxic substances can attack and destroy the cancer lump.

Mushrooms and antitumor activity

There are many who have taken mushrooms favorably as they believe there is anti-tumor activity in the mushrooms. Let us think how the cancer develops. I think liver cancer may be easily explained. Hepatitis progresses to cirrhosis. And cirrhosis progressed to liver cancer on most cases. This is what we believe.

My guess is liver cancer has been started already during hepatitis. We diagnose as hepatitis because there is tiny number of cancer cells which we can't detect by any tests. Hepatitis means lots of heat in the liver. But when the liver turns to cold through cirrhosis, the diagnose becomes the cancer. I already mentioned that mushrooms have warm property. I believe there is a potential to facilitate hepatitis to liver cancer if the patient takes mushrooms on hepatitis. Mushrooms taking may deteriorate hepatitis instead of anti-cancer. However the cool body person may be very helpful due to warm property of mushrooms. When the liver is really cold, the warm nature of mushrooms is going to neutralize the cold stagnation and help the cancer. The anti-tumor activity of ginger, curry, onions, and peppers has the common which produces heat.

CONCLUSION

Even though something bad may be useless, it is true the reality is truly useful in the end. On the other hand some known as very good foods may be harmful to the human body. I believe to impose the theory that the food containing certain substances or ingredients must be unconditionally good for certain symptoms. The best approach is to face head with western medicine and oriental medicine and try to find each other's strength. In this way we can help and provide many people truly informative health.

FEMALE MENOPAUSE

Average age in the past was 50 years old. It has been reported that menopause comes at the age of 49 years old. When the menopause arrives in the past, it is the signal that has been a time to die soon, but now the average age is 80-90 years old meaning they have to live more than 30-40 years. Unless you understand and prepare well, you may be very troubled.

I mentioned already there is a cycle in the age on the subtitle "why do woman marry to man who is older than the woman?" It is the best state in the 28-35 years old. After 35 years old physical body becomes downhill gradually. The age of 42 years old enters the menopausal step slowly.

Form this point on, women experience all kinds of discomforts from various parts of the body. Then the menopause comes at the age of 49.

We may say menopause is painful time for women. But it is not all women suffer during menopause. What I am saying now is not accurate statically. One third of women doesn't experience this menopausal pain or don't understand friend's complaints. It is just like a mild cold passing by to them.

One third of women suffer very much. They don't satisfy their husband and even children. If the husband touches her on the night at bed, her nerve becomes on alert. Even though she understands her husband's libido, it is hard to withstand lower abdomen tingling. There is no one who understands her in the family. The only word is at best that everyone suffers as they get older, but why you show off more than others. This is not the comfort, rather make her angrier. Children need her care any longer now and are away from her and are with their friends only. The husband's position still is recognized socially, but she thinks back what she has done so far. Even though she has devoted her life for her husband and children, no one cares about her. All factors sink her feeling causing depression. When she looks at the mirror, her skin firmness sags and unwanted wrinkle lines are all over her face. This is a very serious illness for women. Some even consider committing suicide. They are scary to lose women's function as well as experiencing menopause directly.

One third is in the middle. This group is not serious like as above, but less serious various symptoms. However there is one interesting fact. Almost all of these groups believe they belong to the worst. As much this menopause period is a very difficult time. Therefore it is necessary to prepare in advance, but not many people do this.

Why do these happen? Western medicine explains by the lack of female hormone. Some symptoms are psychological change, sudden hot flash without a warning making fever and cold sweating, night sweating making a whole body covered by sweat, heart palpitation, forgetfulness, hearing difficulty, tinnitus, sleeping disorder, dizziness and hot symptoms on hands and feet.

Oriental medicine defines Yin deficiency. Hormone also belongs to Yin by oriental medicine, but Yin is not limited to hormone only. Let us think the reason one by one.

1. Sudden hot flash

This phenomenon is to correct the balance of yin and yang. Our body must be balanced between yin and yang. It is most desirable that yin and yang are 100 each. However while we get older, the balance may be off: for instance, yin is 60 and yang is 80. If Yin represents the cold and yang does the warmth, there is the difference of 20. The body tries to release 20 to make the balance. You may experience sweating when you are hot. When the body release 20 of warmth abruptly, the adjustment may be required just like the wave of water or seesaw causing fever and cold sweat. Some has to open the window even in the cold winter when this sudden hot flash, even though other family members suffer with cold temperature.

2. Facial flushing

We have two kidneys, one represents kidney yin and the other is kidney yang. Facial flushing happens as kidney yang is greater than kidney yin. This happens usually on cheek bones changing to red color.

3. Night sweating

This means sweating during sleep. This also happens as yin is less than yang.

THE BEST METHOD

The best answer is to fill the lack of 20 in the above example. If you release the excessive yang of 20, the aging process may go on quickly. I don't believe hormone replacement is not the only answer. The reason is as follows.

1. One patient who is a deaf came to the clinic by driving. I asked a question how she drove the car without hearing the any sound. She answered she can sense the danger with unusual sensation on her skin when other car honks. This means the body has another kind of potential we don't know. Even though we have that potential at the birth, we don't use all functions properly as some function is depressed by another function. But if necessary the body can develop and regain the lost function. In other words we try to go back to the puberty when we don't need the secretion of the hormone.

2. North Korean armed agents came down to the South Korea in 1968. One captured agent testified as he was trained in the mountain and dig the grave and stayed inside the

grave, he could distinguish the smell of animals or human beings. Even the baby at the birth can tell the smell of mother, we lost this kind of ability as we don't use it properly. Therefore it is desirable to wake up the potential.

I cannot describe the detailed method for waking the sleeping ability or potential. My guess is to improve the function of kidney yin and kidney yang. This is because estrogen may belong to kidney yin and progesterone may belong to kidney yang. Artificial hormones are produced in the body, so side effects are unavoidable. The only sleeping potential would minimize the side effects and be able to avoid the uncomfortable life.

It is highly recommended to exercise regularly and eat various vegetables as well as eating more fish and beans. I recommend the tea of ge gen and sheng ma. The most desirable one is taking acupuncture treatments and oriental medicines. I have seen many middle-aged women who took these treatments and enjoy the normal life. Oriental medicine consists of filling the lack of yin and yang for kidney.

The next important thing is the marital relationship. We know the fact an adolescent who talks with parents a lot and well taken care of has less tendency of losing the track. Menopausal period may belong to the fall, so the conversation is very important between couples. Husband's warm conversation and love will help a lot to overcome menopausal depression.

OBESITY

Many people try to lose weight. It is very difficult. It is almost the level of the war. But the war with flesh is not easy as we think.

Western medicine uses diet pills for mainly reducing the appetite. If using more than 3-4 months, side effects must be concerned. After taking pills, some experience heart palpitation, anxiety, dry mouth, and night sweating. Some are banned due to the severe side effects.

There is a pill to inhibit the fat absorption. Some patients believe this pill works excellent observing the oil floating on the toilet bowl. However as this is an artificial method, nutritional imbalance will be resulted. If you replace it with a high-fiber diet or medicine, it will be cheaper and desirable in nutritional level.

The liposuction treats only symptoms, but doesn't treat the cause and go back to the old state again.

Western medicine began to suggest a lot of chicken breast instead of red meat as the problem is on fat. Another theory follows such as carbohydrates rather than fat must be reduced. The new theory is these days to increase protein in order to increase muscles. All these theories is to tell how difficult treating the obesity. One thing is the truth is not changed.

It is very simple to lose weight. Let me introduce the formula. There is no one who doesn't know this formula.

Total intake of calories-total calories consumed=remaining calories

If the remaining calories are greater, it is gaining the weight. If the remaining calories become minus, it is to lose weight. If the remaining calories are zero, the status remains the same. The only way to lose weight is to reduce the total intake and increase total consumption. This means to eat less and exercise more eventually. There is no one who doesn't know, but most who have tried couldn't practice.

Reasons I have been interested in obesity

I read an article about the obesity in November, 2011; one Australian famous acupuncturist. He charges 8899 Australian dollars per person. The losing weight is 5-10Kg in a month. He provides oriental medicines and teaches Qi Gong. Even though he charges 15 times more than his master, he cannot accept new patients for the next 5 months. I believe he makes a fortune. I want to challenge him. If other acupuncturist can do, why can't I make it happen as long as I give my effort on this issue?

Approaching difference between men and women

Men think the first about exercise for the diet. Meanwhile women come to mind to eat less. Exercising belongs to yang and men belong to yang. Foods belong to yin and women belong to yin. This shows how subtle combination of yin and yang. It is always desirable to balance yin and yang. If anyone chooses his favorite, the success would be in half.

The difference in the form of men's and women's obesity

Men's type is mainly like an apple. This form is pop-up around the navel. Women's shape is like a pear. Western medicine explains this different shape with male and female hormones. I have thought this matter for a long time in order to describe this by oriental medicine.

We can say fat means flesh more than normal. There are two types of fat; one is soft and the other is solid. This is due to damp and heat of spleen based on the constitution. The person with more damp than heat has soft flesh and the person who has more heat than damp has solid flesh. Soft flesh is a little easier treatable as the function of spleen is off. The problem is solid flesh. This means flesh and fat together. We have to understand the exact cause in order to solve the problem. We sometimes heard "I don't eat meat at all, but I do have fat. I don't know why." It is understandable gaining on the body fat due to greasy foods such as meats. So we have to find the reason of getting fat even on without greasy foods. Some interprets it may be to put a lot of vegetable oil, sesame oil etc. on vegetables. However it is well-known fact that the liver produces triglycerides through carbohydrates.

The spleen is responsible for flesh as well as damp-heat. Organs have a tendency to give away to other organs if the burden is more than capable. We call this action the over control. In another words, when spleen can't manage by itself, all burdens will be given to kidney which spleen can control easy. As far as unwanted portion is concerned, kidney doesn't want to keep. Kidneys try to send back to spleen, but it is not possible. So kidneys try to send the unwanted portion to heart that spleen can control.

Kidneys are organs to generate essence. Kidneys send away damp-heat to heart with essence, Essence means hormone and bone marrow. Many know that the semen of a man is commonly tacky. The fat is the combination of damp-heat and essence in my opinion.

THE SHAPE OF APPLE AND PEAR

Why are apple-shaped obese men and pear-shaped obese women? Men belong to yang and women belong to yin. This means men have more yang and women have more yin. Yang has a tendency to rise and yin has a tendency to sink. All organs composed of yin and yang. Kidneys also have yin and yang and are composed of kidney yin and kidney yang. Men have more yang going up higher. Women have more yin going up less. That's why different shapes are made between men and women.

When women come to an age of menopause, they become to an apple-shaped obesity. Menopause means the female hormones are gone as we understand. Of course female hormones belong to yin of yins. I believe you are enough to understand why.

SEVERAL CONDITIONS LOSING WEIGHT

1. After illness or the loss of appetite; spleen deficiency
2. Long time diarrhea; spleen deficiency
3. Using ephedra; increasing heartbeat
4. Thyroid hyperactivity; increasing heartbeat
5. Hot places; increasing heartbeat and sweating
6. Spicy foods; increasing heartbeat and sweating

As you see from the above example, we may use spleen function weaken and heartbeat increase. These can be done by acupuncture and oriental medicines, but I don't recommend the loss of appetite by artificial way.

CONDITIONS OF GAINING WEIGHT

1. White flour foods
2. Sweet foods
3. Meat
4. Overeat
5. People who live on cold places need more fat.
6. Alcohols cause to retain more water temporary.
7. Salty foods cause more water retaining.

Personal experience

1. There was a time I love to walk slowly. While I hold my two hands in the back, I walk slowly and hate excessive moving. My weight was 176 pounds. I experienced a little breathing difficulty. I don't have to perspire at all as I can turn on air conditioner in the car and the work place is always cold in the summer.

    I had a chance to cut down the tree branches. In the mean time I smelled a strange nasty smell. I found it came from my body. All these happened were because waste products are piled up in the body as I don't have a chance to sweat.

2. I used to eat just before going to bed as I had to work late and became hungry. As soon as I stopped eating before I go to bed, my weight began coming down.

3. Everyone knows eating more causes overweight. I believe there are lots of people who gain the weight when you went to buffet restaurant. As the price is expensive, we used to eat a lot more than usual. We regret after seeing the weight scale on the next day.

4. Let me introduce my trick when I was young. It is the Treasure Island's hunt. There are many entrances and a flag in the center. Only one entrance can lead to the flag. So most of us failed many times and had to start a new entrance. When I compete with friends, I used to win often. The method is simple. I start from the flag to the entrance.

We can use this method to handle the obesity learning from mistakes. According to my experience, certain foods contribute gaining weight; ice cream, white flour foods and meats.

WHAT IS THE REASON BEHIND?

1. I like ice cream so much which is sweet. Maybe that's why my personality is sweet. But the spleen is related with sweet taste. I mentioned already if the spleen is overburdened, the spleen sends away to other organ. That is the reason to avoid the sugary foods.

2. Avoid foods made with white flour. I am going to give an example to explain about this. We apply paint or wallpaper to decorate the rooms. We need the paste to apply the wallpaper to the wall. Do you know how to make the paste? Add water to white flour and mix well and heat it up. The white flour turns to the paste.

   Now let us think how white flour is changed in the body. The representative foods are noodles, bread and pizza. When we eat these foods, we also get along with water, soda, and soup. The stomach is the hot organ called the middle burner in oriental medicine. The stomach mixes foods well making like porridge and sends to the small intestine in order for small intestine to absorb all nutrients.

   The inside of small intestine has many villas to increase the surface area. If the surface of small intestine looks like plastic pipe, the surface area would be not much. If the paste covers all these villas, villas can't absorb all nutrients available. Not only the paste blocks absorption, but also remains in the intestine. Beer belly shape will be formed. The paste is sticky that can hold other foods causing more weight.

3. Lack of nutrients causes obesity. For example heart is supposed to require magnesium. The heart sends a signal to the brain magnesium is required. The brain sends a signal to the stomach hungry making us eat foods. The stomach asks the heart to be quiet. The heart waits expected magnesium. Until When? The answer is until

necessary magnesium arrives. There are two conditions. If there is no magnesium, magnesium for the heart can't be expected. Even though there is magnesium, and if the intestine is full of pastes, it can't be absorbed. If other unnecessary calories come into the body. It is natural to gain weight.

4. The next one is meat. Typically there is almost no fiber and plenty of fat. Fiber is the substance scraping unneeded one like sponges and sending out of the body. On the other hand the meat contains lots of fat making the fat store in the body. As everyone knows, once stored, it is difficult to take it out.

5. There are surprisingly many people who don't have energy without eating meats. Meat comes from animals. Animals belong to yang. So we can conclude these people are lack of yang energy. One method is to take herbal medicines for a supplement yang.

    However, most meats have lots of fats. You may experience to steam or boil beef short-ribs. Look inside the pot next days. You may find the thick layer of white fat. Everyone would ask themselves they must eat this fat, especially beef fat.

    We must wash this pot with hot water and detergent, otherwise the fat remains the same. No matter how much cold water passes, the greasy sink remains the same. Then how do you get rid of the fat entered in the body? Drinking the hot water is possible, can we drink detergent?

6. There are two types of oil; hardening oil and unconsolidated one. Fresh lard left on the room temperature remains as unconsolidated. It hardens only inside of refrigerator. One interesting fact is the oil of omnivore's animals doesn't get hardened at the room temperature. These animals are pigs, ducks and chicken etc. However grass eating animal's oil is

hardened at the room temperature; beef, goat, lame and rabbit etc.

GENERAL FACTS

1. There is a tendency that the people in the tropical area are relatively thin and in the arctic regions are fat. Most tribes in Amazon River are not fat, but people in cold climates need more fat to combat against the cold. That's why most diet methods are recommended with warming.

2. As mentioned above, cold water can't do the job to remove the fat inside of the sink. Housewives already know this fact well by the experience that the hot water running does the job. Therefore it is very highly recommended to eat warm foods; warm personality foods and drink warm water.

APPROACHING METHOD BY TCM

1. There is a concept of five zhang and 6 fu in the oriental medicine. The obesity is the result of excessiveness or weakness and coldness or hotness of particular organs. This means if one supposed cold organ becomes warm, we have to make it cold. The organ supposed to be warm must be changed to warm. The weak organ must be changed to strong. The excessive organ must be removed the excessive portion to make it in balance. Without doing these and just with diet and exercising means the cause remains the same and treats symptoms only causing y0-yo to return to the original position. The diet and exercising alone are good for the short term effect, and so yo-yo happens as this is lack of treating the deeper cause. This can be done of course by acupuncture and herbal treatments.

2. One of the reasons of obesity is the fat absorbed in the small intestine moves to the heart. This fat passes to the

capillaries through the artery. Some fat can't return to the vein and remain on the skin. The solution is to melt the fat by the warming methods.

3. There may be minimal fat between intestines. But if the inside intestine becomes full of fat, there is a possibility osmotic activity from the inside of intestine to the outside where there is less fat. This may be one of the reasons of accumulating the fat between intestines. One method is to remove the fat by warming the fat between intestines and the other is to remove the fat inside intestines. This may enable opposite osmotic activity from the outside intestine to the inside one in order to make the balance in and out.

4. We must observe the organ transformation to prevent yo-yo. When we exercise, you can see the veins in the skin may appear on the surface of the skin. This is due to the heat. The heat has a tendency to expend and the cold has a tendency to contract. If the expansion is greater than the contraction, the volume of the organ would be larger. If the volume becomes larger, you may feel hungry even though you take the same amount of foods. This means you have to take more foods. This will cause the probable obesity again. Therefore it is right to make warmer to make the fat melt, but we have to make certain organ to be cold to prevent yo-yo.

5. Western medicine becomes successful on many cases by making smaller stomach with a surgery or using a clip. Of course there are adverse effects. This method can be achieved by oriental medicines by making cold stomach. The coldness can make the contraction and eat less to avoid yo-yo. When we try to make this in hasty, there are side effects such as chilling feeling on the stomach or even diarrhea.

6. But it is not necessary to make small stomach unconditionally. Some suffers with poor digestion most of

times. As this happens because of weak stomach function, it is better to make the stomach warm to enable spleen Qi vaporization. Many in this case suffer with edema and the flesh is usually soft. In this case gastrectomy may cause serious health problems. This is the reason we should not consider only one method.

7. The adjustment of other organs as well as the stomach is also required. For example gallbladder has a function to secret the bile against greasy foods and reduces the absorption of oil. If there is no bile, the oil may accumulate in the body. This would follow the increase of cholesterol. This is the reason why the bile is generated and secreted well.

8. It is the same with small intestine and large intestine. The expansion or contraction is required depending on the individual symptoms to prevent yo-yo.

9. Exercise to increase the metabolism

    a. Most of movements help the metabolism. The problem is everyone knows the exercise is good, but can't keep it. According to several studies the effect of exercise begins 20 minutes after. Therefore it is necessary to take 30-50 minutes of exercising.

       There is "Biggest loser" program in TV. I don't know how many hours of exercising, but looks like very harsh exercise. However how can many people invest such harsh exercise in the reality working in the workplace? Actually many people go back to the original state after losing the weight. It is usually better off to do moderate exercise than radical movements.

    b. After exercising we experience sweating. We have to understand what the sweat is. Sweat belongs to body fluid out of body composition such as qi, blood, body fluid and essence. The sweat is the purpose of dissipating the heat in the body. However it is desirable to sweat the proper amount, but the excessive sweating would be harmful for the body. The torture level of exercising is harmful. Have you seen the basketball playing in TV? They run back and force without a rest and perspire a lot. These players should live longer theoretically, but players don't live longer than general population. Therefore the forehead is wet by sweating or if 5-10 minutes of sweating since it breaks out is better off stops exercising

c. There are two major types of exercising. One is the radical movement and the other is the slow movement. The radical movement causes the sweat faster and a lot. The slow movement causes the sweat slowly and a little. The young people may be acceptable with the radical movement, but as we get older, the exercise like walking is more desirable.

d. It is important where you exercise. The outdoor is more desirable than the indoor. It is better where there are more trees. Why? There is more oxygen where more trees are. Some research shows the result that effects in the park are double.

10. The goal is 10% of body weight for the first three months. You may give up or easily fail if you set the goal too high. You may achieve this goal within two months or four months. The important point is to set up the goal achievable. As soon as you achieve the goal, you set up another 10% again. The reason is based on not too easy or not too difficult. This method is based on psychology.

Most people are happy with just 5-10% losing weight. One interesting fact is from the moment we find to lose the weight; the amount of foods is reduced.

11. What should we eat?

  1. Recommended foods have fewer calories but contain more nutrition with satiety feeling. You may find so called witch soup in the internet. Someone says that this soup is called witch soup as the taste is so bad. Ingredients are cabbage, bell peppers, carrots, onions and tomatoes etc. These are mainly consisting of vegetables. Some add chicken breast. I suggest changing a little bit not to get tired of the same foods only.

  2. Dark colors are better for the body in many cases. Oriental medicine calls five colors; green, red, yellow, white and black. You may replace the black with purple color.

  3. There are many theories about the snacks, but let me introduce my experience. It is difficult to endure when I become hungry. Until I eat something to conquer the hunger, all my attention are on over the hungry and I can't do anything. If we eat cookies on the hunger, we are going to fail to escape from the obesity. Oriental medicine old book suggest foods enabling to conquer the hunger on small amounts. One of them is jujube which we can get easily. Potatoes or sweet potatoes are good. If unbearable, eat low-calories. But any snacks are forbidden right before the night sleep. I already mentioned on the biometric time of body-organ.

  4. Obesity is not to lose weight for a short period of time, but should be managed for a life time. We need

wisdom to choose fishes over the meat even though we love meat.

5. We must be happy about eating meat just once a week. The reason is explained already.

6. There are two types of foods we eat. One is to eat when we are hungry. The other is not able to resist the temptation over the emotional eating. Emotional temptation is over certain foods like pizza, ice cream and chocolate etc. We have to eat more than the required amount on sudden time instead of any given time. Most regret after this emotional eating. This is related with women menstruation. We must treat this issue before treating the obesity.

   Eating when we are hungry is desirable over the emotional eating. We have to be careful not to overeat and follow the method described above.

7. When we get stressful, we try to eat more than usual to relieve the stress in many cases. It is necessary to find your own method to reduce the stress and even obesity.

WESTERN AND ORIENTAL MEDICINE

I know one man who is 80 years old. He is so healthy and able to clean the gutters with a ladder across the roof. So I asked him how he manages his health. His nephews advised him not to take any medicines except Bayer aspirin and vitamins and minerals. His nephews worked as secretary of State department of Health in USA.

The reason is Bayer aspirin was made 100 years ago by Pfizer whose side effects are the minimum. Not only works well as pain killers, but also prevents heart disease and many other good functions.

Vitamins also have been over 80 years. Almost no side effects have been reported except vitamin A which is not soluble in water. All medicines are safe and proven as they are used for a long time.

Tremendous capitals are required to develop a new medicine, so it is difficult to start from the beginning. After being developed, a lot of time and budgets are required for clinical trials against animals. Another ten years takes clinical trials for humans. If this trial is passed, FDA approves.

The meaning of the approval is the benefit is much greater than the risk.

There are a few cases of unexpected side effects since the medicine has been marketed, even though very few side effects are reported in the beginning. As soon as the report of side effects comes out, the withdrawal of medicines but also the lawsuit that got harmed by the side effects will follow. Huge amount of money is paid for the lawsuit.

In general western medicines have fast healing effects and more side effects. Most western medicines are made chemically. As humans come from the nature, our body cells can take care of most edible foods produced naturally. However body cells may confuse how to take care of chemicals. This confusion shows as side effects in my opinion. Many side effects are written with small letters on most medicines. If not listed properly, the pharmaceutical company may be sued, so many side effects are supposed to be written.

In the oriental medicine the body is viewed as a microcosm; a part of nature. Most herbs are from roots, bark, leaves, stems, flowers, seeds, and saps etc. Special stones or a part of animals are used occasionally.

Oriental medicine's healing is slowly effective compared with western medicine, but side effects are far less relatively. Oriental medicines are proven more than at least 500 years based on oriental medicine treasure. All formulas are tested by many intelligent herbalists. After they try the same formula into many different ways, they discovered the most effective and safe ways.

For example jie geng (radix platycodonis) is the herb to carry all ingredients into lungs. This is the action of leading something to certain spot. Western medicine uses this method these days, but this method is already used 500 years ago written by the book of oriental medicine treasure. I strongly believe if we apply these formulas into western medicine, healing effects are great. But there are two problems.

The first thing is enormous capital requiring FDA approval. The second thing is these medicines can't get patents as these information are already known, even though lots of money invested. Without patents it is difficult for capital recovery, so many companies don't take risks as any other companies can copy.

We don't consider this harsh reality of the oriental medicine, but believe the oriental medicine is unscientific. This concept is just like ancient people are not wiser and smarter than the present people. For example it is well known that radishes help better digestion since ancient times. Experiments with modern science, radishes contain diastase helping better digestion. This kind of debate is meaningless just like which one is the first, chicken or egg. However it is our fault of present oriental medicine's practitioners as we have not developed further. It is also difficult to deny the theory and practice of oriental medicines.

I heard there is a dispute over new natural medicine based on oriental medicine between western medical doctors, pharmacists and oriental medicine practitioners. As this medicine is made of pharmaceutical way, western medical doctors have prescriptive authority, but oriental practitioners are not allowed to prescribe. Upon the complaints of oriental practitioners that this new medicine belongs to the oriental medicine and is invaded, no one wants to involve and solve this delicate issue. I believe this is because no solutions make everyone happy. Let me ask a question. Most western doctors claim that the oriental medicines are unscientific. My question is if only the form is changed by them, the medicine becomes scientific.

It looks to me a just greedy of trying to take a bigger piece of a pie than to think of the health of patients.

Helicobacter pylori and Gastritis

One patient has suffered with poor digestion, heart burn and abdominal pain and went to see the doctor. The MD thought this may be gastritis or peptic ulcer symptom and suggested the gastroscopy examination to make sure. Helicobacter pylori were detected from the biopsy, so the patient was on medication as MD explained H pylori cause gastritis. The patient didn't notice much for two days on the medication. As time passed by, the patient became uncomfortable feeling and suffered heart burn, headache, dizzy and diarrhea. He went through this trouble. He felt to go to the hell on his money. This is the first time of this kind of experience on his life. He got the second biopsy and was told that H pylori are still there, so he needs more medication.

He asked me there is any other way in the oriental medicine. I answered him this is a piece of cake with a little exaggerating. He was delighted, but couldn't believe it.

Stomach acid is very strong digestive fluid like hydrochloric acid. The hydrochloric acid is able to make a fire on touching the paper in the laboratory. Nobody assume that any bacteria can grow at this condition. These are found in the last part of stomach; pylori. Western medicine believes these cause gastritis, even stomach cancer, but some believe everyone has some H pylori meaning annihilation may be not desirable.

Western medicines use the antibiotics to devour bacteria in the body. On the contrary there is no concept to kill in oriental medicine. The oriental medicines try to create the environment for bacteria to hate to stay. What kind method do I use?

Growth of bacteria requires the proper temperature. For example the foods left in the outside room are spoiled fast in the summer time. But the foods kept in the refrigerator remain almost unharmed. Now this concept goes on H. pylori. The fact this bacteria can survive in the strong acid is this bacteria must have very cold nature. Therefore more heat makes a better environment for H. pylori. This means as gastritis makes better environment for the growth of H. pylori, not as H. pylori cause gastritis.

To treat it as the first step, Chinese medicine is required. This oriental medicine has the following properties. Cactus that grows in the desert has the cold properties as I mentioned already. The easy way to kill the cactus is to move to the cold North Pole area. It is very simple. Does this make sense to you?

Acupuncture treatment on this case would be supplemental to make the imbalance between yin and yang. Oriental herbal medicine is absolutely necessary to treat H. pylori. In addition gastritis or stomach ulcer will be treated naturally at the same time.

IS IT HEALTHY TO LIVE WITH LAUGHTER ALWAYS?

"Rejoice always" is the words in the Bible. When I came across this passage, this verse was so good, so I try to live this way. While I pray, I ask the Lord that I may live this way and try to live this way.

Dr. Sugwan Hwang who created a joyful life passed away with acute septicemia at the age of 67 years old. Many felt awkward with his death including myself. He claimed if we live with laughter, we can have longevity without any diseases. Many agreed and laughed upon his lecture. Considering the average life expectancy of man over the age of 76, Dr. Hwang had failed to fill up the average age. Is this a little bit strange? I have never heard his lectures as I don't agree with his idea.

There was a famous writer and broadcaster who tell audiences to have positive mind as a happiness evangelist. But she chose to commit to suicide. Even though I don't suffer her chronicle disease, I do understand a little bit through treating similar patient. Considering that patient came out of pains, I hope she could try to find other therapists with more hopes. I really hope words and actions are in perfect harmony.

I usually advise young acupuncturists to be a role model as far as health concerned. If the patient comes to treat obesity and finds a practitioner is heavier than the patient, who is going to get the treatment by that practitioner? And the patient comes to stop smoking and finds the practitioner smokes. Who wants to get the necessary treatment from him? Therefore acupuncturists must be a role model in health. Even though it is impossible to maintain perfect health status, it may be possible to show better outer appearance. That's why I think seriously about health issues and make the effort to find the fundamental reason that everyone can understand.

일소일소 일로일로(一笑一少 一怒一老):This means when we laugh once, we become young once. And when we become angry once, we get old once. Everyone heard when we laugh, the blessing will follow. Happiness and rejoice produce the endorphins. Dr. Sanggoo Ahan caused a sensation about endorphins and everyone knows about endorphins. However the effect of endorphins lasts about five minutes. If endorphins may treat pains like morphine, the patient should continue to rejoice. But this is impossible in the reality.

Human beings and most vertebrates have nine glands making endocrine system. Nine endocrine glands to secrete hormones are hypothalamus, pituitary, adrenal, thyroid, parathyroid, gonad, thymus, the islets of Langerhans and pineal glands. I interpret we need all hormones; not more than necessary or less than necessary. If we try to emphasize or seek one thing, our body will lose the balance. Let me explain an easy example. If men have lack of semen and difficult erection, most men become depressed very much.

As I am an acupuncturist, I love to interpret by oriental medicine theory. This theory emphasizes the balance. Let us think about tastes. Our tongue can distinguish sour, bitter, sweet, spicy and salty. This means we have to take all five tastes or flavors to become healthy. Most of us like sweet, spicy and salty tastes, but don't like sour and bitter. Particularly hates bitter taste. This causes illness. Many people know oriental herb medicines are bitter. As the illness comes from lack of bitter taste foods, the bitter taste medicine is required so to speaking. Old saying is good advice bothers ear and medicines are bitter in the mouth. Do you understand why oriental medicines have bitter taste, now?

I believe the bitter taste has an important role to make bile. When the bitter comes into the body, our body accumulates and processes it by many various courses and stores at the gallbladder. When the fatty foods come into the body, the bile comes out and resolves the oil not to absolve in the body and prevents obesity. In case of lack of bile our body can't do the decomposition against the fat. Even though the bitter taste has an important role in the body, we try to be away from the bitter taste. Then we become sick and the bad health would be followed.

I believe this taste principle should apply the same way into emotions.

Oriental medicine define human being has seven emotions; joy, anger, sadness, worry, depression, surprise and fear. I believe we are better off to use all these emotions properly. When we stress only one emotion, this may cause harmful for the health. Everyone is easy to understand being happy on happy moment. However being sad on sadness and being angry on anger could be better off for the health.

We tears on sorrow. When our beloved parent passes away, we tear spontaneously. Some comforts that parents went to the heaven where there is no sorrow and worry, only happiness exists and asks not to be sorry. Even though we understand this fact and try not to be sorry, but tears flow down. This is natural. However we can't see and talk them when I want to see and talk. Until I go to the heaven, we cannot see each other and must be separated. That's why we cry with sadness by the pain of separation. Many families immigrated to the United States cried because of breakup. The United States 30-40 years ago was a heaven compared with Korea without an exaggeration. But many families spilled tears while leaving Gimpo Airport. This kind of grief is quite natural one and we should not suppress in order not to harm the health. Of course too long sorrow is not recommended.

Those who are engaged in the sales or serve a lot of clients can't get angry. As we know a customer is a king. Even if angry and unfair, the only thing they can do is to endure or suppress. This causes depression. Some cry over the anger how pity situation it is for them. These tears may cool down a roaring fire providing the balance in the body. We also know no tears cause glaucoma due to increased intraocular pressure. When tears come down upon sorrow, you may expect lower eye pressure.

Oriental medicine treasure wrote that practitioner made the patient angry and treated the patient. "In your anger do not sin"[a]: Do not let the sun go down while you are still angry according to Ephesians 4:26". Most explain being angry is sin, therefore do not be angry. However my interpretation is we can be angry, but this anger must be forgotten before we go to bed. The reason is simple. It is extremely desirable not to get mad, but this is impossible for human beings. But we can try to forgive and forget and reconcile before we go to bed. I believe this is more realistic for us.

In the past we emphasize IQ as we believe the good brain means success. However we also emphasize EQ is important as well as IQ. That is right. Everyone understands emotions the oriental medicine talks about. But we emphasize too much only on joy, so most emotions are dried up. When someone is in grief, it is better to comfort and help others. This is more desirable for me and others.

I saw an article whose subject was "The optimistic person die earlier". I read this article with a curiosity and that makes sense to me. The point is the optimistic person doesn't go to doctors due to their personality. This leads finding the problem at later stage and the person can't get the treatment on time.

When we are sick, we must laugh. And we must try to do laughing. The reason is all other emotions are at peak except laughing. Therefore we must laugh in order to make the balance in emotions.

In general occasions, we would be better to use all different seven emotions to maintain for the better health.

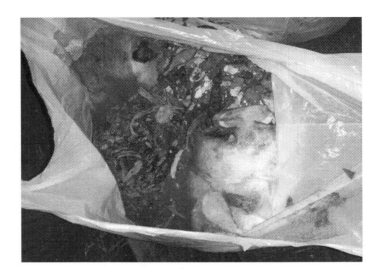

Fungus grows to begin at where plastic bag and left over herb meet. This means in coincidence of cancer growth that cancer cells can grow well where there is no oxygen.

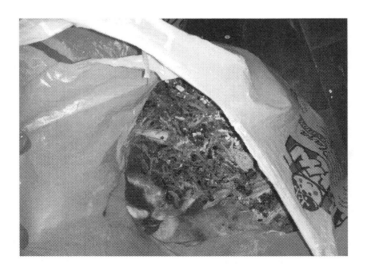

The author's website is

www.acupunctureforpains.com/acupuncture_helps_pain.html

You may find lots of useful information on this website.

If you want to be a friend in the Facebook,

You can look for **Chan Hur** or **Answers with Acupuncture**.

If you ask me questions, I will answer you as long as I have a time for that.

Author's other books

	Eyeglasses	$5000
Save	Toothache for	$2500
	Tinnitus	$4500

http://bookstore.authorhouse.com/Products/SKU-000554364/
Save-5000-for-Glasses-2500-for-Toothache-and-4500-for-Tinnitus.
aspx

About the Author

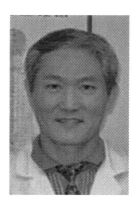

The author pursues the practical thing than a theory. Economy is to study how to be rich in a short sentence. If so, the richest man in theory must be a professor in economics. However most professors do live comfortably, but they are not the richest person.

Mr. Anthony Robinson said that if you want to be a best in a certain field find the best and copy him. While I study in the TCM School, I try to find a best acupuncturist. It had taken a year to find a true master to me. I bought his books and seminar materials and studied his books. This process has made me one of Korean 4 needle specialists.

I could develop some unique approaches that guarantee eczema and acne treatment to be healed within one month. Most claim they are the best, but maybe only one who is me provides money back guarantee. If I don't treat within a month, I treat next month on me. If I still don't treat as promised, I will return the money paid. Is there any more practical way than this?

This book explains strong and weak aspects of Eastern and Western Medicines and advises whom patients must see at the certain condition.